The Essential Guide for Patient Safety Officers

Second Edition

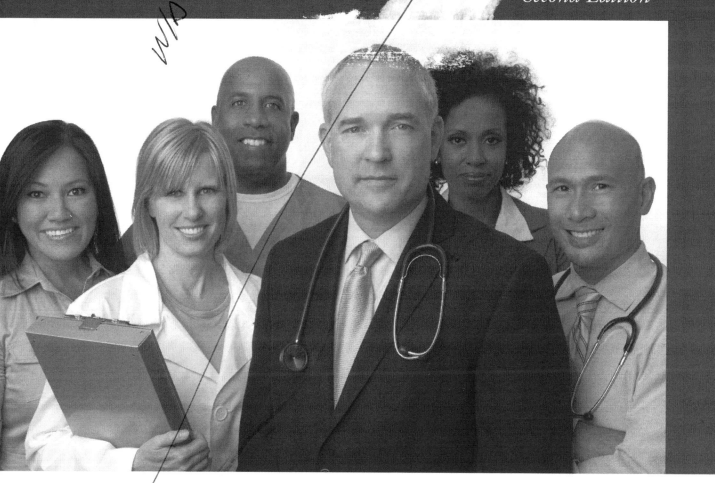

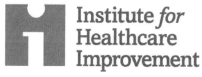

Joint Commission Resources

Edited by
Michael Leonard, MD
Allan Frankel, MD
Frank Federico, RPh
Karen Frush, BSN, MD
Carol Haraden, PhD

Foreword by
Gary S. Kaplan, MD

Institute *for* Healthcare Improvement

Senior Editor: Steven Berman

Senior Project Manager: Cheryl Firestone

Manager, Publications: Lisa Abel

Associate Director, Production: Johanna Harris

Executive Director: Catherine Chopp Hinckley, MA, PhD

Joint Commission/JCR Reviewers: Lynne Bergero, MHSA; Jorge César Martinez, MD; Christina Cordero, MPH, PhD; Sherry Kaufield, MA, FACHE; Ana Pujols McKee, MD; Paul vanOstenberg, DDS, MS; Deborah Nadzam, PhD, RN, BB, FAAN

Joint Commission Resources Mission

The mission of Joint Commission Resources (JCR) is to continuously improve the safety and quality of health care in the United States and in the international community through the provision of education, publications, consultation, and evaluation services.

Joint Commission Resources educational programs and publications support, but are separate from, the accreditation activities of The Joint Commission. Attendees at Joint Commission Resources educational programs and purchasers of Joint Commission Resources publications receive no special consideration or treatment in, or confidential information about, the accreditation process.

The inclusion of an organization name, product, or service in a Joint Commission Resources publication should not be construed as an endorsement of such organization, product, or service, nor is failure to include an organization name, product, or service to be construed as disapproval.

This publication is designed to provide accurate and authoritative information in regard to the subject matter covered. Every attempt has been made to ensure accuracy at the time of publication; however, please note that laws, regulations, and standards are subject to change. Please also note that some of the examples in this publication are specific to the laws and regulations of the locality of the facility. The information and examples in this publication are provided with the understanding that the publisher is not engaged in providing medical, legal, or other professional advice. If any such assistance is desired, the services of a competent professional person should be sought.

Joint Commission Resources, Inc. (JCR), a not-for-profit affiliate of The Joint Commission, has been designated by The Joint Commission to publish publications and multimedia products. JCR reproduces and distributes these materials under license from The Joint Commission.

The Institute for Healthcare Improvement (IHI) (www.IHI.org) is a leading innovator in health and health care improvement worldwide. An independent not-for-profit organization, IHI partners with a growing community of visionaries, leaders, and front-line practitioners around the globe to spark bold, inventive ways to improve the health of individuals and populations. IHI focuses on building the will for change, seeking out innovative models of care, and spreading proven best practices. Based in Cambridge, Massachusetts, with a staff of more than 140 people around the world, IHI mobilizes teams, organizations, and nations to envision and achieve a better health and health care future.

Printed in the USA 5 4 3 2 1

Requests for permission to make copies of any part of this work should be mailed to
Permissions Editor
Department of Publications and Education
Joint Commission Resources
One Renaissance Boulevard
Oakbrook Terrace, Illinois 60181 U.S.A.
permissions@jcrinc.com

ISBN: 978-1-59940-703-6
Library of Congress Control Number: 2012950204

For more information about Joint Commission Resources, please visit http://www.jcrinc.com.

CONTENTS

FOREWORD

In reading this second edition of *The Essential Guide for Patient Safety Officers,* I was struck by the progress that we've made in understanding patient safety since the first edition's publication in 2009. The work described in the book reveals growing insight into the complex task of taking care of patients safely as an intrinsic, inseparable part of quality care. To do this we need to create a systematic, integrated approach, and this book shows us how to do it.

This new approach not only addresses our own desires to do the best we can for our patients but also reflects the influence of external forces such as demands for greater transparency and accountability. The impact of health care reform through the Patient Protection and Affordable Care Act[1] on health care providers is far-reaching, including increasing emphasis on the following:

• Quality metrics—to enable payers (the government, employers, and patients) to identify hospitals and other health care organizations that are providing the best outcomes and safest environments for care.

• The patient's experience—as the government's hospital Value-Based Purchasing program links a portion of the hospitals' CMS (Centers for Medicare & Medicaid Services) payments to performance on the 27-item HCAHPS [Hospital Consumer Assessment of Healthcare Providers and Systems].[2,3] Safety certainly influences patients' perceptions.

• Cost control and efficiency—which are critical for the well-being of health care providers, the overall health care system, and, indeed, the entire economy. For example, providers can receive incentives from government programs such as the Medicare EHR (electronic health record) Incentive Program (including the meaningful use criteria),[4] which motivates medical centers to use EHRs that improve efficiency, accuracy, and safety.

This book outlines several crucial elements of safe care delivery. One is the full engagement of health care leadership in improving patient safety. Organizations emphasize and pursue what leaders, by their example, believe is important. Executive management must lead and be seen to lead improvement work, and this naturally includes patient safety improvement. As a CEO myself, I can attest to the truth of this. And, as Chapter 1 points out, leaders must not only lead the effort, they must "learn that the science of reli-

ability is essential to their role. They must understand and accept the science behind this work and expect others—including other leaders, physicians, and staff on the front line—to learn about it."[(p. 3)]

Physician leadership is an important part of leadership commitment. An organization that reforms around physicians but does not make them a part of the team will not succeed in the long run. As Chapter 1 reminds us, organizations with stronger physician leadership have been shown to be more successful in delivering change.

This book points out that a culture of safety is not a culture that seeks to blame individuals when things go wrong. Humans are not individually capable of the sustained awareness and attention required for perfect patient safety. On the other hand, as Chapter 10 tells us, the human factor is crucial to a successful system. The human operator is the "one system component that has the capability to resolve the unanticipated forms of failure that emerge in complex systems."[(p. 111)]

Technology alone is not the answer but is a crucial part of the systems we need to develop. Achieving the promised benefit, while avoiding the risks inherent in health information technology (HIT), will require us to integrate our use of technology into "human factors, cognitive engineering, and the team-based concept to have maximum effect. Applying HIT to the most complex human endeavor of health care will require the development of new approaches for the design, development, implementation, and optimization of the overall system of care, not just information technology."[(p. 113)]

The effective team is a central aspect of safe care, complementing and using technology intelligently. The very diversity of education, outlook, and experience found on teams that communicate effectively (which is so important to collaboration—Chapter 6) is their strength. Each member will see things a bit differently; together they will see the whole.

As discussed in Chapter 9, sometimes overlooked in the movement to create teams are patients and families, who make good partners in the care delivery process. Their insights and experience add invaluable knowledge to our improvement efforts. Patients and families are increasingly well informed and want be involved in care decisions. They also have the right to understandable information, not only about their care and treatment, but also about outcomes and results. We don't yet have a simple way to provide meaningful comparative data, but, as stated, such transparency is part of the reform effort.

When an adverse event occurs or is only narrowly averted, we must be straightforward in disclosing it to all concerned. Disclosure is the right thing to do—and can be viewed as another way to engage patients and their families in care (Chapter 8). It helps begin the coping process, it greatly helps in identifying and repairing systems issues that led to the event, and it may actually improve public perception of the organization.

I am pleased that Chapter 12 covers two improvement approaches, both developed in industry—the Model for Improvement and Lean, which has been gaining ground in health care more recently.[5] The chapter provides a good overview of how Lean improvement efforts work. We have been taking the Lean approach, based on the Toyota Production System, since 2002; we call it the Virginia Mason Production System.

Now, all our collective efforts to improve patient safety will fail if we don't recognize that this endeavor entails remaking and transforming health care as we know it. That means rethinking our assumptions and accepted truths, attitudes, and practices. Keeping patients safe is a leading indicator of how we are doing in this transformative work.

—*Gary S. Kaplan, MD*
Chairman and Chief Executive Officer,
Virginia Mason Medical Center, Seattle

REFERENCES

1. US Government Printing Office. H.R. 3590: The Patient Protection and Affordable Care Act. Jan 5, 2010. Accessed Oct 29, 2012. http://www.gpo.gov/fdsys/pkg/BILLS-111hr3590enr/pdf/BILLS-111hr3590enr.pdf.

2. US Department of Health & Human Services, Centers for Medicare & Medicaid Services. HCAHPS: Hospital Care Quality Information from the Consumer Perspective. Accessed Oct 29, 2012. http://www.hcahpsonline.org/home.aspx.

3. US Department of Health & Human Services, Centers for Medicare & Medicaid Services. Summer 2012 *HCAHPS Executive Insight* Letter. 2012. Accessed Oct 29, 2012. http://www.hcahpsonline.org/executive_insight/.

4. US Department of Health & Human Services, Centers for Medicare & Medicaid Services. Welcome to the Medicare & Medicaid EHR Incentive Program Registration & Attestation System. Accessed Oct 29, 2012. https://ehrincentives.cms.gov/hitech/login.action.

5. Furman C, Caplan R. Applying the Toyota Production System: Using a patient safety alert system to reduce error. *Jt Comm J Qual Patient Saf.* 2007;33(7):376–386.

CONTRIBUTORS

EDITORS/AUTHORS

Michael Leonard, MD
Co-Chief Medical Officer
Pascal Metrics
Washington, D.C.
Adjunct Professor of Medicine, Duke
    University
Durham, North Carolina
Faculty, Institute for Healthcare
    Improvement
Cambridge, Massachusetts
michael.leonard@pascalmetrics.com

Allan Frankel, MD
Co-Chief Medical Officer
Pascal Metrics
Washington, D.C.
Faculty, Institute for Healthcare
    Improvement
Cambridge, Massachusetts
allan.frankel@pascalmetrics.com

Frank Federico, RPh
Executive Director, Strategic Partners
Institute for Healthcare Improvement
Cambridge, Massachusetts
ffederico@ihi.org

Karen Frush, BSN, MD
Chief Patient Safety Officer
Professor of Pediatrics
Clinical Professor, School of Nursing
Duke University Health System
Durham, North Carolina
karen.frush@Duke.edu

Carol Haraden, PhD
Vice President, Institute for Healthcare
    Improvement
Cambridge, Massachusetts
charaden@ihi.org

AUTHORS

Mary Ann Abrams, MD, MPH
Iowa Health System
Des Moines, Iowa
abramsma@ihs.org

Barbara Balik, RN, EdD
Faculty, Institute for Healthcare
    Improvement
Cambridge, Massachusetts
Consultant, Pascal Metrics
Washington, D.C.
barbara.balik@pascalmetrics.com

Doug Bonacum, MBA, BS
Vice President, Quality, Safety, and
    Resource Management
Kaiser Permanente
Oakland, California
doug.bonacum@kp.org

Jeffrey P. Brown, MEd
Senior Cognitive Psychologist
Cognitive Systems Engineering Group
Cognitive Solutions Division
Applied Research Associates
Fairborn, Ohio
jeffbrown@arar.com

David C. Classen, MD, MS
Chief Medical Information Officer
Pascal Metrics
Washington, D.C.
david.classen@pascalmetrics.com

James Conway, MS
Adjunct Faculty, Harvard School of Public
    Health, Boston
Principal
Pascal Metrics
Washington, D.C.
jbconwaywoburn@gmail.com

Andrew P. Knight, PhD
Assistant Professor of Organizational
    Behavior
Washington University
St. Louis
knightap@wustl.edu

Robert C. Lloyd, PhD
Executive Director of Performance
    Improvement
Institute for Healthcare Improvement
Cambridge, Massachusetts
rlloyd@ihi.org

David Munch, MD
Senior Vice President and Chief Clinical
    Officer
Healthcare Performance Partners, Inc.
Gallatin, Tennessee
dmunch@hpp.bz

Gail A. Nielsen, BSHCA, FAHRA, RTR
Director of Learning and Innovation
Leading the Center for Clinical
    Transformation
Iowa Health System
Des Moines, Iowa
Faculty, Institute for Healthcare
    Improvement
Cambridge, Massachusetts
nielsega@ihs.org

Sarah Pratt, MHA
Vice President, Client Services
Pascal Metrics
Washington, D.C.
sarah.pratt@pascalmetrics.com

Roger Resar, MD
Senior Fellow, Institute for Healthcare
    Improvement
Cambridge, Massachusetts
rresar@ihi.org

Doug Salvador, MD, MPH
Associate Chief Medical Officer and Patient
    Safety Officer
Maine Medical Center
Portland, Maine
salvad@mmc.org

Natasha Scott, MSc
Director of Scientific Instruments, Applied
    Science
Pascal Metrics
Washington, D.C.
natasha.scott@pascalmetrics.com

Jackie Tonkel, BSBA
Vice President, Consulting
Pascal Metrics
Washington, D.C.
jackie.tonkel@pascalmetrics.com

Introduction

CREATING A ROAD MAP FOR PATIENT SAFETY

Michael Leonard, MD; Allan Frankel, MD; Frank Federico, RPh;
Karen Frush, BSN, MD; Carol Haraden, PhD

Anna Rodriguez—a 27-year-old mother of young twins—enters a preeminent teaching hospital for arthroscopic knee surgery on a Tuesday morning after a holiday weekend. The surgery department has a full schedule, with both elective and emergency surgeries scheduled.

Eileen Page, a registered nurse and 20-year veteran of the hospital, preps Ms. Rodriguez in the preoperative area. Per the organization's protocol, Ms. Rodriguez is supposed to receive prophylactic antibiotics one hour before her surgery. Because it is approaching 45 minutes before Ms. Rodriguez's scheduled surgical start time, Ms. Page is in a hurry to give the preoperative antibiotics. Busy with another patient as well, Ms. Page has dozens of procedural steps she must perform to ready both patients for surgery, and she inadvertently overlooks checking the medical record for allergies. Unfortunately, Ms. Rodriguez is allergic to certain antibiotics, including the ones that Ms. Page is about to administer. Buried in the many pages of the medical record is a note about a significant systemic reaction to antibiotics, but no one has noted Ms. Rodriguez's allergies in a prominent place where Ms. Page could easily be reminded.

Because she is in a hurry, Ms. Page tries quickly to explain to Ms. Rodriguez what she is doing. Ms. Rodriguez is from Venezuela and does not speak English well. Ms. Page does not speak Spanish, so communication is sketchy at best. The Spanish-speaking nurse on staff is busy attending to another patient, and Ms. Page is trying to move Ms. Rodriguez quickly into surgery so the surgery schedule will not be delayed. Organization leadership has repeatedly stressed to frontline staff the importance of adhering to the surgery schedule—cases must start on time. In fact, management closely tracks the percentage of cases that start on time and continually pushes to improve it.

As Ms. Page begins to administer the antibiotics, Ms. Rodriguez becomes agitated because of her lack of ability to

communicate clearly. Although Ms. Page notices the agitation, she assumes Ms. Rodriguez is just nervous before her surgery.

Approximately 45 minutes after receiving the antibiotics, Ms. Rodriguez is brought into the operating room (OR). The surgeon is anxious to get started and curtly calls the OR team together to begin surgery. As the surgery begins, the OR staff notices that Ms. Rodriguez's vital signs are abnormal, and she appears to be in respiratory distress. The team is unclear as to what is happening. The surgeon and anesthesiologist work to stabilize the patient while one of the circulating nurses checks the medical record. Ms. Rodriguez suffers cardiovascular collapse and is ultimately resuscitated but suffers significant severe neurologic injury.

After reviewing the medical record, the team realizes the nature of the problem. Ms. Page is devastated. The media swarms onto the campus of the medical center, asking difficult questions, but do not receive what they perceive as satisfactory answers from the leaders of the institution. Clinicians and hospital administrators don't interact with Ms. Rodriguez's family in a way that makes them feel that they understand what happened, so they retain an attorney to represent them. The media stir up public outrage about this tragic mistake. Leadership in the organization begins to look for someone to blame for the incident, and Ms. Page seems like a good candidate.

Eventually, hospital leadership goes before the press and public and commit to eliminating medical errors in their facility and improving safety. They hire a consultant, launch some safety initiatives that target medication errors, and feel confident their work is making a difference. However, the root causes of the event that occurred in the OR are still present in the organization: lack of communication, lack of teamwork, lack of patient involvement, lack of reliable processes, lack of organizational emphasis on safety and reliability, and the inability of the organization to continuously learn from its mistakes. Although the implemented safety initiatives may improve medication safety in the organization for a short time, they serve only as a Band-Aid for a deeper, more long-term problem.

What if this operating room scenario or one like it occurred in your organization? Would the response have been the same? Does your organization and its senior leadership value and commit to a culture of safety? reliable systems? teamwork and communication? Is the accountability system in your organization structured to protect the hardworking nurse like Ms. Page, who inadvertently makes a mistake because of a series of system errors? Or is it designed to identify fault and place blame? Does your organization have a systematic approach to responding and learning when errors occur? Does your organization have an open and honest disclosure process? Are patients involved in their care? Do they have a voice within the organization? If your answer to any of these questions is "no," you are not alone. However, you are also nowhere near where you need to be in providing safe and reliable health care.

ALL WORK AND NOT ENOUGH GAIN

In the United States and elsewhere, hospitals and health systems are struggling to improve quality, reduce the current unacceptable levels of harm, engage physicians in improving safety, and deal with regulatory and operational pressures. For many care systems, the current cost structure and dynamic is not sustainable. Quality and safety are increasingly tied to financial incentives and disincentives. The recent Institute of Medicine (IOM) report, *Best Care at Lower Cost*,[1] notes that more than a decade since the IOM's report *To Err Is Human*,[2] we have "yet to see the broad improvements in safety, accessibility, quality, or efficiency that the American people need and deserve."[1(p. ix)]

Recent studies assessing harm and adverse events indicate that roughly one in three hospitalized patients in the United States have something happen to them that you or I wouldn't want to happen to us; with 6% of hospitalized patients being harmed seriously enough to increase their length of stay and go home with a permanent or temporary disability.[3] A majority of these events are judged to be avoidable or ameliorable—meaning that the outcome could be changed if the care team was aware quickly and took action to resolve the issue.[4] Yet it has been estimated that only 14% of adverse events are reported into reporting systems,[5] which reflects the woeful lack of systems designed to proactively

seek near misses and adverse events for learning and improvement. We have also come to appreciate that high levels of harm occur in ambulatory care, particularly in diagnostic errors and adverse medication events. More than 50% of medical malpractice claims stem from outpatient care.[6]

The substantial gap between the kind of care that is often provided and safe and reliable care occurs despite the best intentions and unflagging efforts of skilled, dedicated practitioners and administrators. There have been some successful individual efforts to address the issue of safety, although much of the work has been fragmented, focused on specific areas only, and not sustained beyond the short term.

ADDRESSING THE ROOT OF THE PROBLEM

The primary reason for the lack of progress is that organizations are not addressing the root of the safety problem. Yes, decreasing error is important, but it cannot happen without an environment that supports a systematic approach to creating and maintaining reliable processes and continuous learning. In other words, before an organization can realize sustained improvement, it must commit to designing reliable processes that prevent or mitigate the effects of human error, and establish a culture in which teamwork thrives, people talk about mistakes, and everyone is committed to learning and improvement. When an organization achieves an environment of reliability and continuous learning, then patient safety becomes a property or characteristic of the organization and, by definition, the organization starts to reduce errors.

MAKING SAFETY AN ORGANIZATIONWIDE IMPERATIVE

So how do you achieve an environment in which reliable processes exist and continuous learning is an intrinsic value? It doesn't happen by just telling employees to try harder to be safe. It requires a systematic approach that addresses the fundamental ways in which providers interact and provide care. Such a systematic approach involves four critical components[7]:

1. A strategy, which focuses on reliability and continuous learning. This strategy represents an organization's basic values and vision as well as its goals.

2. A structure, which consistently supports the strategy and helps integrate it into the accepted way of doing business. Such a structure builds the appropriate framework,

designates the appropriate resources, and defines the reporting relationships that effectively support the strategy.

3. An environment or culture that supports the structure and ensures the proper execution of deliverable outcomes to meet strategic objectives, such as reduced error and enhanced patient safety

4. Clear outcomes and associated metrics that are visible, both internally to the people doing the work and externally to the market and the public. These outcomes and metrics help drive consistent improvement within the organization.

A ROAD MAP FOR SUCCESS

The Essential Guide for Patient Safety Officers provides a road map to enable health care organizations to create the necessary strategy, structure, environment, and metrics to improve the safety and reliability of the care they provide. On the basis of the Institute for Healthcare Improvement's Patient Safety Executive Development Program—a synthesis of patient safety experts' collective experience—and our experience and that of the other contributors, each chapter focuses on a different stop along the map, as follows:

• The Role of Leadership—Effective leadership is critically important at all levels of a health care organization. High-performing organizations teach, embed, and reinforce effective leadership behaviors. It is also essential to have systematic processes that support dialogue, learning, and improvement between frontline providers and senior leadership.

• Assessing and Improving Safety Culture—Safety culture provides valuable insights as to what it feels like to be a unit secretary, nurse, physician, or other caregiver at a clinical unit level. Feeling valued and having the psychological safety to speak up and voice concerns and learn from errors all have a tremendous impact on the quality of care and the social dynamic among caregivers. Safety culture is measurable and can be deployed as a powerful mechanism to engage caregivers in positive behavioral change.

• Accountability and the Reality of the Human Condition—Error and avoidable harm are prevalent in health care today, and fear of blame and punishment is a major obstacle to learning and improvement. High-performance organizations are characterized by fairness and high degrees of accountability. Applying a consistent and fair algorithm to evaluate errors and adverse events that is rein-

forced by senior leaders is essential for learning and improving care.

• Reliability and Resilience—Consistent, measurable processes of care delivery are foundational to achieving the desired process and outcome measures. Habitually excellent organizations do the basics very well, which provides a foundation for innovation and learning. High degrees of variation, in which clinicians "do it their way" without transparent metrics, leads to inconsistent care and high rates of harm.

• Systemic Flow of Information—Few health care organizations have built process to support robust dialogue between the wisdom of bedside caregivers and senior leaders who are trying to navigate a complex operating environment. Clinicians experience basic system failures every day that are frustrating and wasteful and that get in the way of optimal care. Capturing and acting on these insights drives better care, improves efficiency, and builds organizational trust.

• Effective Teamwork and Communication—Progressively more and more literature is now showing that effective teams deliver better care, to the benefit of not just patients but caregivers. Building teamwork across an organization is intentional work, not just a project, making the difference between sustainable value and "flavor of the month."

• Using Direct Observation and Feedback to Monitor Team Performance—There is a robust science used in numerous industries to observe performance and the associated team behaviors, and provide feedback for learning and improvement. Observation and feedback have been used quite effectively in medical simulation and clinical care environments to provide insights that help drive better care.

• Disclosure—In the aftermath of patient harm or unintended consequences, patients and providers need to be able to talk openly and honestly. This is a learned skill; fear of looking incompetent or getting in trouble often precludes dialogue that is both candid and respectful. Open, honest disclosure needs to be an organizational priority.

• Ensuring Patient Involvement and Family Engagement—We are learning more and more about the benefits of delivering care that is truly centered on the patient and family. Organizations that engage the voice of the patient, listen and learn and incorporate these insights into continually improving the care process will not only deliver better care but are more likely to be successful in a rapidly changing health care environment.

• Using Technology to Enhance Safety—Health care is a sociotechnical process, with skilled humans continually interacting with technology and information systems. Technology can deliver much value if carefully assessed, implemented, and monitored, but if not, technology can negatively affect work flow and increase the risk of patient harm.

• Measurement Strategies—Improvement requires measurement and continuous learning associated with specific skills that are teachable and must be embedded throughout the organization. Measurement strategies are an essential, foundational component for the delivery of safe and reliable care.

• Care Process Improvement—A sample of the many practical methodologies that have been successfully applied within health care to drive improvement and positive change is provided. Key to all are the studying of the process targeted for improvement, the identification of areas of risk and waste, and the determination of opportunities for improvement.

• Building and Sustaining a Learning System—Caring for patients is an extremely complex process, as reflected by the many interrelated topics addressed in this book. A practical framework is essential to support a systematic approach to increasing the quality and safety of patient care. In the absence of such a framework, it is not possible to sustain continual learning and improvement. Successful safety work is not a series of projects but the integration of work so that it is visible, measurable, and sustainable. That is the overall aim of this book.

SUMMARY

This book is designed to help anyone in an organization improve the safety of care provided to patients—from the patient safety officer (or other senior leader) to frontline staff who are charged with improving the provision of care. It details the critical steps involved in enhancing patient safety throughout an organization and ensuring the reliability of care. A full reading gives a clear understanding of what is involved in creating and sustaining a culture of safe and reliable care. You will be armed with tips and tools from other organizations that have engaged in these efforts to apply to your own organization.

Some of the concepts discussed within this book may seem simple in theory, but they can be quite challenging to implement, and dependent on organizational support and a strategic approach to improvement. It takes a commitment from all levels to systematically drive this work and achieve success. By incorporating the different elements discussed in this book into everyday work, organizations can continuously improve, enhance, and achieve patient safety.

The editors acknowledge their colleagues who continue to teach us and advance their understanding of safe care delivery; Richard Bohmer, Donald Kennerly, Gary Kaplan, Aileen Killen, Lucian Leape, Tami Minnier, Paul Preston, Bob Wachter, and Michael Woods deserve special mention. The editors thank Steve Berman, Jane Roessner, and Kathleen B. Vega for their assistance in the development and writing of this book.

REFERENCES

1. Smith M, et al., editors; Committee on the Learning Health Care System in America, Institute of Medicine. *Best Care at Lower Cost: The Path to Continuously Learning Health Care in America.* Washington, DC: National Academies Press, 2012.
2. *To Err Is Human: Building a Better Health System.* Washington, DC: National Academy Press, 2000.
3. Classen DC, et al. 'Global Trigger Tool' shows that adverse events in hospitals may be ten times greater than previously measured. *Health Aff (Millwood).* 2011;30(4):581–589.
4. Levinson DR. *Adverse Events in Hospitals: Medicare's Responses to Alleged Serious Events.* Report No. OEI-01-08-00590. Washington, DC: U.S. Department of Health & Human Services, Office of Inspector General, Oct 2011. Accessed Oct 29, 2012. https://oig.hhs.gov/oei/reports/oei-01-08-00590.pdf.
5. Wright S. *Few Adverse Events in Hospitals Were Reported to State Adverse Event Reporting Systems.* Report No. OEI-06-09-00092. Washington, DC: US Department of Health & Human Services, Office of the Inspector General, Jul 19, 2012. Accessed Oct 29, 2012. https://oig.hhs.gov/oei/reports/oei-06-09-00092.pdf.
6. Lorincz CY, et al. *Research in Ambulatory Patient Safety 2000–2010: A 10-Year Review.* Chicago: American Medical Association, 2011. Accessed Oct 29, 2012. http://www.ama-assn.org/resources/doc/ethics/research-ambulatory-patient-safety.pdf.
7. Frankel AS, Leonard MW, Denham CR: Fair and just culture, team behavior, and leadership engagement: The tools to achieve high reliability. *Health Serv Res.* 2006;41(4 Pt 2):1690–1709.

Chapter One

THE ROLE OF LEADERSHIP

Doug Bonacum, MBA, BS; Karen Frush, BSN, MD;

Barbara Balik, RN, EdD; James Conway, MS

Governance and leadership are ultimately responsible for quality and safety.[1,2] The most important factor in achieving safe patient care at a system level is overt, palpable, and continuous commitment from organization leadership to set an aim, create a strategy, establish a structure, and foster an environment that encourages, supports, and requires safe and reliable care. Such a strategy, structure, and environment cannot exist without the collaborative commitment of senior administrative leaders, boards of directors, and physician and nursing leaders. Performance improvement and enhanced safety may occur in small areas or individual units through a grassroots approach, but improvement cannot be sustained or spread throughout an organization without the active participation of organizational leaders.

Partnering with formal and informal leaders, particularly senior executives and the organization's board of directors, to achieve safer care is an essential part of a patient safety officer's role. This chapter will assist you and your leadership partners in achieving safer care outcomes.

As discussed in the Introduction, achieving safety is not a one-time or short-term effort. Major progress requires a multifaceted leadership approach,[3] implemented and revisited over time, which includes activities such as assessing a culture for safety,[4] ensuring the technical and cognitive competence of each individual, responding to data, striving for high reliability,[5] embracing transparency,[6] fostering communication and teamwork,[7,8] setting meaningful goals,[9] and sharing outcomes.

The following are eight essential leadership steps to achieve safe and reliable health care[2]:

1. Establish, oversee, and communicate system-level aims starting at the governance and executive leadership level.
2. Identify harm, design and implement improvements, and track/measure performance over time.

3. Assess the culture for safety and act to close any gaps.
4. Understand the science of improvement and reliability—strive to be a high-reliability organization (HRO).
5. Foster transparency.
6. Create a Leadership Promise.
7. Engage physicians and nurses, especially those in executive and formal leadership roles.
8. Hire for what you aspire to become.

ESTABLISH, OVERSEE, AND COMMUNICATE SYSTEM-LEVEL AIMS

Leaders must establish a portfolio of system-level aims aligned with the organization's mission, vision, and values. These aims form the foundation for communicating what is important, creating operational and administrative alignment, and facilitating accountability at each level in the organization. The level of performance expected in system-level aims is often not what the organization presently views as possible (for example, eliminating health care–associated infections), requiring new ways of thinking and acting that stretch beyond the comfort level of those in operations.

The effective leader listens to the concerns and opinions of those who feel unreasonably stretched by the pursuit of aggressive system-level aims, and then clarifies the roles of those individuals and provides the resources necessary to foster success. Measurement systems that track the pathway to performance are established, and the leader routinely reviews progress along the pathway, transparently communicates about that progress, and consistently holds the organization accountable for its progress. Achievements are celebrated and deficits are studied and remedied.

An example of a "SMART" system-level aim that has been transformational for many organizations was the Institute for Healthcare Improvement's 100,000 Lives (5 Million Lives) Campaign,[10,11] which benefited from having

Specific, Measurable, Achievable, Relevant, and Time-bound goals. For each topic area or "plank," the campaign provided how-to guides, which described key evidence-based care components and how to implement the interventions and recommended measures to gauge improvement.[11] Leaders who accepted the 100,000 Lives challenge answered the call of "if not now, when?" and "if not you, who?" and in doing so, inspired their organizations to achieve great things. The effective leader listens to the concerns and opinions of those who feel unreasonably stretched; sets clear expectations; provides any needed resources, including education and training; and establishes ways to measure performance. After goals are established, effective leaders are steadfast in expecting accountability.

IDENTIFY HARM, DESIGN AND IMPLEMENT IMPROVEMENTS, AND TRACK/MEASURE PERFORMANCE OVER TIME

Tightly coupled with the leader establishing and communicating system-level aims, there must be a cascading set of measures that align from front office to front line. Leaders call for data associated with these measures to be current and transparently posted to increase accountability for performance, promote dialogue during rounding and day-to-day operations, and get the patient/family member more engaged and involved in his or her own care.

At the board level, important measures are typically large-scale system outcome measures such as mortality, global rates of harm, readmission rates, and serious safety events. At the frontline level, measures must also include those that are grounded in process reliability. For example, the board may want to know the "days since the last health care–associated infection" as a measure of the system-level aim, "Eliminate health care–associated infections." The service-line aim is to eliminate catheter-related infections across the geriatric service, and the geriatric intermediate care unit's frontline aim is to reduce catheter-associated urinary tract infections.

ASSESS THE CULTURE OF SAFETY AND ACT TO CLOSE ANY GAPS

Creating a healthy organizational safety culture typically requires a shift in the way that clinicians, patients, administrative staff, and leadership view the health care organization

and their respective roles in it. For the organization to be successful, leadership must encourage, support, and drive change from both the top down and the bottom up. The common and inaccurate belief that a health care organization is a collection of smart, hard-working individuals trying really hard to provide safe care must be challenged. Effective leaders understand and promote the evidence-based view that a health care organization is a complex set of teams of professionals, patients, families, and leaders who work together to systematically provide the most effective care in the most efficient way.

One of the first steps in changing a culture involves assessing the culture in its current form at all levels. Team- and unit-level data are essential to this endeavor. As discussed further in Chapter 2, cultural assessment involves looking at a variety of data—both quantitative and qualitative—that measure culture, including staff perceptions of safety, teamwork, management, stress recognition, and job satisfaction.

Other data that can also reveal information about your organization's culture, include reports or lack of reports about potential safety issues that come into a spontaneous reporting system; analyses or lack of analyses of near misses; and stories of concerns from caregivers gleaned during rounding processes, such as Executive WalkRounds[12] and/or direct observation in care settings.[13] As described in Chapter 2, organizations have recently begun looking for and establishing correlations between unit-level outcomes and culture data. Not surprisingly, units with high teamwork and safety climate scores tend to perform better on almost all measures that matter, including efficiency, patient injury, and staff turnover rates.[14] Sharing these results with staff provides additional motivation to change.

While these activities are discussed further in later chapters, they are mentioned here to reinforce the point that leaders must commit to using a variety of types and sources of data to learn about an organization, its culture, its strengths, and its weaknesses. A prioritized action-oriented plan can then be developed to deal with any weaknesses and measure performance moving forward. As recently reported, the 9 ICUs (out of a total of 23 ICUs) in 11 hospitals in the state of Rhode Island that completed action plans to address culture survey results later demonstrated higher improvement rates in five of the six survey domains.[15] Leaders must become experts in looking for trouble and be open to seeing problems, particularly those that may exist beyond a leader's primary attention. Avoiding the temptation to judge problems as rarities is difficult but very important.

Effectively interacting with data involves not only analyzing and responding to them, but also considerable effort in ensuring that the most useful data are collected. It is important to note that more data are not necessarily better and can just get you lost in the analytic process. The key is to select focused, actionable data, and then develop focused and actionable performance improvement plans to address deficits.

The clearer your organization can be on what data will be most relevant to assess the organization's culture, determine areas of improvement, and drive action, the better.

UNDERSTAND THE SCIENCE OF IMPROVEMENT AND RELIABILITY

Health care is a complex endeavor. The processes of health care can and should be designed to anticipate and mitigate human error and ensure that processes occur the way they are designed and achieve the outcomes they need to achieve. In other words, processes must be designed so they are reliable. As discussed in Chapter 4, designing reliable processes that support safe practice and mitigate human error involves critical assessment of current processes, careful planning, and the use of the science of reliability (*see* page 33).

Leaders must learn that the science of reliability is essential to their role. They must understand and accept the science behind this work and expect others—including other leaders, physicians, and staff on the front line—to learn about it. Most health care leaders and professionals did not learn the science of reliability in their professional education, thus it is likely they may not even know it exists. Even so, it is the responsibility of leadership to understand and apply reliability science to the daily work of the organization. What this means practically is that leaders should require (1) time-trended data to be used to assess process performance over time; (2) work flows to be simplified and standardized through application of performance improvement strategies, such as the Model for Improvement (*see* Chapter 12, page 125), coupled with the application of rapid-cycle "small tests of change"[16] (*see* Chapter 4); and (3) that when an individual cannot adhere to standard work, the issue and relevant circumstances be brought back to a process owner for dialogue and learning. To accomplish this, leaders must commit to organizationwide training on these concepts.

While reliable processes are one component of a reliable organization, there are other aspects involved in embedding reliability at the cultural level, an activity that is essential to working toward functioning as an HRO.

At their most basic level, HROs experience fewer accidents despite typically operating in "risky" and complex environments.[17] The operational attributes of HROs that allow them to perform at this level, as defined by Weick and Sutcliffe, are (1) reluctance to simplify, (2) deference to expertise, (3) preoccupation with failure, (4) sensitivity to operations, and (5) commitment to resilience.[5]

Examples of HROs in which the aforementioned attributes are apparent include commercial aviation, naval nuclear power, aircraft carrier operations, hazardous chemicals manufacturing, and aeronautical industries. Such industries achieve reliability because they actively seek to know what they don't know, design systems to make available important knowledge that relates to a problem to everyone in the organization, learn in a quick and efficient manner, aggressively avoid organizational arrogance or the belief "errors cannot happen here," train organization staff to recognize and respond to system abnormalities, empower staff to act, and design redundant systems to catch problems early.[18] In other words, an HRO expects its organization and its subsystems, regardless of how reliably they are designed, to fail, and the HRO works very hard to avoid known sources of failure while preparing for unexpected failures, so that the organization can minimize both the frequency and impact of future failures.[5]

Those looking to migrate their organizations toward HRO status should begin by clarifying the leadership role involved, committing to regularly assessing stories that provide a window to understand the organization's culture—reviewed annually—and implementing a set of expected behaviors, activities, and initiatives that other organizations have used to successfully drive change. Many of these behaviors, activities, and initiatives are described throughout this book.

FOSTER TRANSPARENCY

Transparency in health care involves openness in communication, the routine production and wide-scale distribution of unblinded performance data, acknowledging and reporting error, offering an apology when harm occurs, defining accountability at all levels in the organization, and committing to system improvement. A transparent organization does not try to hide mistakes, but acknowledges that errors occur and works to fix the systems that ultimately cause those errors. Such an organization accepts that it is not perfect, and continuously works to identify areas of improvement.

A culture is transparent only if its leaders define, role-model, and cultivate that transparency. There are many ways to do this, including the following:

• Openly discuss failure. Talk about, discuss, and analyze issues, errors, and risks with frontline staff, medical staff, patients, families, and the public.

• Establish an environment of psychological safety in which everyone is comfortable speaking up. Each individual, and what he or she has to say, must be treated with respect at all times, and disrespectful actions can't be tolerated by leaders. Psychological safety is essential for open communication to occur, for when individuals believe that they or their suggestions are being criticized, they will cease to contribute to the discussion. (*See* Chapter 6 for further discussion about psychological safety.)

• Share data—both good and bad—on performance with frontline staff, medical staff, patients, families, and the public. When appropriate, leaders should establish an expectation that staff members produce their own trended and annotated data to demonstrate their ability to improve and sustain performance over time. When data relate to a process improvement project, leaders should routinely confer with the process owners concerning progress in and possible barriers and obstacles to meeting goals. When implementing new initiatives, it is critical to share the results and show if a process does, in fact, improve patient outcomes and increase efficiency. To sustain physician and staff involvement in improvement, they must believe that improvement is being realized and the process does work. For example, when implementing a new insulin protocol, data, including graphs, should be provided to show the extent of possible reductions in episodes of hyper- and hypoglycemia. To reinforce a sense of commitment, people need to know that their work and efforts are worthwhile. We must recognize their achievements and specially highlight their good work all the time.

• Provide avenues for feedback, such as Executive WalkRounds[12] (*see* Chapter 5). Respond to feedback with communication and examples of improvement in a timely manner to encourage further feedback.

• Develop leadership skills across the organization for transparency, so the ability to consistently share data, safely learn from failures, and reinforce an accountability model is a foundational organizational property at all levels.

• Be consistent when responding to close calls and adverse outcomes with a leading edge focus on what happened and not who did it. Leaders should establish an accountability system to differentiate between system issues, human error, and at-risk behavior (for example, a violation of safe practice) and apply that system consistently across the organization regardless of outcome.[19,20] (*See* Chapter 3 for a further discussion of accountability.)

• Although the following points are not directly related to transparency, active work in these areas is important in supporting a transparent culture:

— Foster teamwork and effective communication across the organization. (*See* Chapter 6 for a further discussion of teamwork and communication.)

— Involve and develop the capacity of all stakeholders in improvement, including frontline staff, medical staff, patients, and families.[21,22] Involve patients in their care through multidisciplinary rounds, transition reports, and eliminating visiting restrictions; talk openly and honestly with patients and families when things go wrong; apologize; and ensure ongoing support for patients and families who have been harmed.[23] (*See* Chapters 8 and 9 for more information.)

Many organizations are fearful of transparency, as they believe it will reveal flaws and increase lawsuits. The concern is that if the organization exposes its weaknesses, people will capitalize on those weaknesses to the detriment of the organization. However, there is research that shows that this is not what typically happens. In fact, being transparent often increases trust with patients and families. When one hospital in the Pacific Northwest was open and honest about a high-profile medical error, the public responded positively to the organization, believing that the organization was working to provide the most appropriate care and, when it failed, was open and honest about it. When Paul Levy, former CEO of Beth Israel Deaconess Medical Center in Boston, openly discussed a wrong-site surgery error on his weekly blog, it stirred a spirited discussion within the medical community[24] but also resulted in appreciation from the public for his openness, honesty, and transparency.

Being transparent also has the benefit of improving employee morale and engagement in improvement efforts. Sharing data about strengths and weaknesses excites and motivates staff to participate in improvement efforts. It reflects a commitment to be candid and continually improve.

CREATE A LEADERSHIP PROMISE

One specific action that organization leaders can do to help verbalize their commitment to transparency and high reliability is to create a Leadership Promise. This is a document that clearly delineates the role of the leader in safety, reliability, and performance improvement. Sidebar 1-1 on page 6 is an example of one organization's Leadership Promise. Compacts between physicians and health care systems can also be helpful in terms of clarifying expectations and increasing joint accountability. In addition, asking all staff to sign a pledge to adhere to specific behavioral performance standards can set a tone regarding the seriousness of the behaviors and facilitate both recognizing excellence and correcting nonconformance.

ENGAGE PHYSICIANS, NURSES, AND OTHER CLINICIANS
Getting Physicians on Board

To transform complex health systems, physicians must be engaged as leaders in their health care settings, in both formal and informal roles,[25] and at the institutional, service-line, and frontline levels.[26] Gosfield and Reinertsen define this future state as "physicians working together systematically, with or without other organizations and professionals, to improve their collective ability to deliver high quality, safe, and valued care to their patients and communities."[27(p. 5)] When physicians share their personal passion, expertise, and responsibility, there is a high likelihood that improvement efforts will be stronger and more accepted as the "way to do the work." Organizations with stronger physician leadership have been shown to be more successful in delivering change.[26]

Without physician engagement, safety improvement efforts will be flawed in their design, have trouble getting off the ground, and/or have difficulty being sustained. Physicians have a huge impact on the quality of care delivered, clinical variation, and resource consumption, not only in their own practices but across the continuum of care experienced by patients.

Effective physician relationships with governance, leadership—including specifically nursing leadership—frontline nurses, pharmacists, patients, families, and others are essential for the consistent delivery of safe, high-quality care. Any changes in the way care is designed and delivered require physician participation and acceptance either as individuals or as a professional body.[27]

Engaging physicians in improvement initiatives has historically been a challenge for physicians and for health care organizations. In the past, physicians were largely excluded from the improvement process. In the division of labor, hospital leaders have viewed performance improvement as their responsibility and that of their administrative, nursing, and other clinical (largely nonphysician) staff. When physicians were consulted, it was often after the initiatives were identified or at the end of a process design. Physicians may serve in unpaid administrative roles in health care organizations, and because of time constraints and their need to focus on their first priority (direct care of patients), they often lack the time, energy, or motivation to get involved in performance improvement initiatives.

In many instances, the quality and safety priorities for health care institutions and physicians have been and continue to be out of alignment. Although many physicians give generously of their time to support their community hospitals, they have little additional time to spare for the organization's quality and safety agenda. When the priorities of the hospital and physicians come into conflict, it can strain relationships, thereby undermining collaborative problem solving and performance improvement efforts.[28]

The challenge, and therefore the solution, to this issue lies in developing and inspiring physician leaders to expand their sense of responsibility beyond individual patients to the health care organization—and its ability to provide better care. The physician culture is largely based on personal responsibility for patient outcomes and contributes to physicians' attachment to individual autonomy. Physicians are taught that "If we work and study hard enough, we won't make a mistake." This leads them to believe that if a mistake does happen, it is their—or some other person's—fault. This cultural element puts physicians in conflict with a now emerging systematic approach to patient care that entails shared, as well as individual, accountability. Physicians often fail to see their role in a larger system, the many components of which may come together to form high-risk situations

Sidebar 1-1. Not on My Watch

Following is one organization's Leadership Promise. It is a written document that organizations can use to help verbalize a leader's commitment to safety and reliability.

I am at the helm of a medical center that intends on providing the safest hospital care in the United States by the end of the year [fill in year]. We will do this by eliminating all preventable death and injury to our patients as we continue to pursue a workplace free of injury to our staff. In partnership with our physician and union leaders, our safety aim is routinely communicated to every employee and physician, and more recently, to our patients.

I actively oversee a three-year plan to achieve our goal that builds off of the great work we've already begun. By *actively oversee*, I mean that I receive monthly progress reports and require corrective action plans to close identified gaps. In concert with this activity, I personally track a small number of hospitalwide patient safety measures that are routinely updated and made fully transparent to our staff and to our members; these measures include hospital risk adjusted mortality, a global harm rate generated by use of the IHI Global Trigger Tool, bundle compliance for bloodstream and surgical site infections, as well as ventilator-associated pneumonia (VAP) and never events.

I have tied our patient safety aim to other hospitalwide initiatives, including improving flow, eliminating workplace injuries to our staff, and improving service. In the process, my CFO has become a true patient safety champion, realizing that safe, reliable care is no accident, and no accident is good for our bottom line. In addition, each member of my senior leadership team is required to cosponsor a patient safety improvement initiative. This helps them better understand the complexity of providing safe, reliable care, and allows them to better connect their activities to our aim.

Each week, I personally spend about four hours on matters directly related to the provision of safe, reliable care. During this time, I:

✔ Conduct Executive WalkRounds and review reports indicating the status of issues that staff have identified during our time together
✔ Review all significant events and sign off on each one with a statement that says I have reviewed the case and that it appears the corrective action plan will significantly reduce the risk of recurrence . . . of course, I'm not the only one who makes this certification, but I am the last one. I also make sure that lessons learned from both our own, and other medical centers' events, are shared with our frontline practitioners. After all, they are the ones who have a need to know.
✔ Spend 10 minutes at new employee and physician orientation to make clear, in no uncertain terms, my views of patient safety and my expectations of them. I also let them know that my door is always open to safety and how they can contact me.
✔ Follow up on reports of unsafe practitioners and make sure that we are not only addressing identified issues of competency, but identifying issues related to collaboration, respect, and organizational values
✔ Visit with our member-driven, patient safety advisory council and hear directly from our members what's concerning them and what's going well
✔ Act as an executive sponsor of improvement initiatives related to eliminating unwarranted variation in work flow and process . . . medicine is complex enough without having eight different ways of doing the same thing.
✔ Review resource requests concerning patient safety that have been denied at lower levels in the organization. I agree with most of the decisions made, but want everyone to understand, the buck stops here with respect to patient safety.
✔ Visit with one of our performance improvement teams on the floor to hear and see specifically how their work is going. We currently have initiatives related to eliminating preventable infection, medication, and birth-related injuries. They are all on 90- to 120-day performance improvement cycles and so I see remarkable progress every week.

By far, the hardest thing I do is to meet with patients/families who have suffered a significant, preventable injury while in our care. It may also be the most meaningful thing I do.

On an annual basis, I ensure that the current state of the organization's patient safety culture is measured. In between, I am driving the creation of a just culture by demanding a brief on every patient safety–related event where part of our response strategy has been to use discipline. I'm all for accountability . . . and to ensuring that our response is "Just."

As more and more patient safety demands are placed on the organization by state, federal, and accrediting bodies, I sponsor a review of our staffing and structure to ensure that we have the resources in place to do what's needed. I periodically update my own knowledge of patient safety and demand that my executive team does the same. This year, [fill in the blank] members of our team are attending the IHI Annual Forum.

As well as I think we generally do here, I recognize that to go from where we are to where we want to be is going to require a relentless commitment on my part to improve patient safety. Only I can productively direct efforts to foster the culture and commitment required to address the underlying systems causes of medical error and harm.

Preventable Death and Injury? Not on My Watch . . . Not in My Region . . . Not in My Organization!

Source: Doug Bonacum. Adapted and used with permission.

that can result in harm to patients. This personal responsibility approach to patient outcomes continues to reinforce a blaming culture.

Compounding this cultural bias, and specifically related to patient safety, is the fact that most physicians rarely see data for the adverse events in which they were involved. Medical staff organizations and hospitals have not historically developed expertise in identifying harm, and even when they do, most physicians do not receive direct feedback on their care.

Fortunately, among physicians and health care leaders, there is a growing and shared understanding that there is too much harm, much of it preventable; there is both shared and individual accountability and responsibility; and the solution lies in collaborative performance improvement efforts and true engagement of physicians in a shared quality agenda.

So how can organizations engage physicians?

Achieving Clinical Integration with Highly Engaged Physicians offers six comprehensive steps to achieve physician engagement: (1) discover common purpose, (2) reframe values and beliefs, (3) segment the engagement plan, (4) use "engaging" improvement methods, (5) show courage, and (6) adopt an engaging style.[27] For example, for "discover common purpose," a key element in engaging physicians is to match improvement goals with things physicians value. Physicians care about initiatives that affect their patients' health outcomes, such as fewer infections, lower mortality, and other indicators of safe care. Like other members of the health care team, they seek to "first, do no harm" and make sure that the care provided to patients is appropriate and effective. In addition to improved patient outcomes, physicians value their time. For most physicians, time is a rare commodity. They are juggling multiple patients with complicated conditions in many settings with multiple payers, and they need to make decisions in a time frame that is at best short. Physicians will embrace change that improves efficiency and saves time for their patients and for them. Processes that result in less wasted time, fewer hassles, reduced bottlenecks and delays, and minimized rework will gain their support. In some cases, the importance of time can trump the importance of patient outcomes. In other words, if an effort improves outcomes but costs more time, physicians, regardless of their motivation, may be unable to comply with the improvement effort. Demonstrating short- and long-term clinical, financial, and service outcomes may be necessary.

Physicians also want to see data. Visions and goals, no matter how captivating, are generally of limited value to them. If organization leadership can show physicians that new processes are making patient outcomes better and giving the physicians more time, then physicians will be more likely to support performance improvement efforts, thus enhancing the probability that such efforts will be successful.

It's important to note that by mirroring organizational performance improvement objectives with those of physicians, your organization does not have to sacrifice its own quality goals. For example, if you pursue better patient outcomes and increased physician time, you decrease length of stay, enhance efficiency, and improve financial performance. In other words, organizational outcomes will improve as a by-product of patient outcomes and time efficiency.

Following are some practical considerations when working to involve physicians:

• Physician quality has historically been associated with peer review, which is generally perceived as a punitive process, not an opportunity to learn. Reframing the conversation as an opportunity to improve the quality of care provided is essential. Teaching about system error and having a model of accountability is key to supporting this cultural shift.

• Physicians enjoy contact with the board of trustees not only as members but as invited guests. Find opportunities to have governance and medical staff meet, not to hear reports but to engage in productive conversations.

• Physicians, like all of us, love to give opinions—create a physician advisory group to do patient safety work. But be ready to shut up and listen. There is no group that will end quicker than one that doesn't lead to action and improvement.

• Formal recognition can play an important role in the life of most physicians and can include celebrations and recognition programs. Recognizing physician involvement and leadership in performance improvement and patient safety can reinforce the importance of physician input.

• Paying physicians less than what they would earn is often acceptable; what is critical is to acknowledge that their time is valuable. Consider paying physicians four to eight hours a month to be "Patient Safety Champions."

- Don't waste their time. Physicians have a strong aversion to "task forces for life." Physicians are very action oriented—they want to see results.

- Physicians respond to clinical data more than opinion. Measure and obtain clinical and survey data that will withstand scrutiny. When the data lose credibility, so do leaders, and recovering that credibility is very difficult. Measure items that physicians have identified as important to them.

- Consistently reinforce the message that effective teamwork is critically important for delivering safe, high-quality care.

- In debates and disagreements, always focus on what's best for patients. That helps anchor the conversations around a common goal.

There is growing evidence that cultural barriers can be dismantled and collaborative practice enabled by appealing to "the better angels" by doing the right thing, by showing the data, and by defining strategy around the patient's needs.[28(p. 58)]

Following the 80/20 Rule to Drive Improvement and Develop Physician Leaders

When trying to engage physicians, it is difficult to work with every physician in the hospital and ensure their comprehensive support and involvement. In all likelihood, 80% of your organization's medical staff rarely steps foot in the hospital. While essential members of your community, these are not the individuals on whom you should initially focus your efforts, unless there is someone with a very special interest. It is the 20% of staff members who spend the majority of their time working in the hospital—the hospitalists, residents, full-time staff, and medical staff members who regularly practice in the hospital—who have a clear, vested interest in improving clinical care. They also are firmly grounded in what works and what doesn't and what should be improved.

Within that 20%, you should identify those individuals who embrace change and value performance improvement. These champions can help colead initiatives, address issues, and generate support and engagement of others. But first, you need to invest in these potential leaders, positioning them for success. Considerable efforts have been taken to understand the key competencies of physician leaders, and organizations should familiarize themselves with them.[29,30]

There are significant barriers to physician leadership; for example, formal systems frequently hamper the development of such leadership, and leadership capability among physicians is not systematically nurtured. Yet perhaps even more important, many clinicians have deeply held beliefs about leadership as "low value" and do not view it as core to their professional identity.[26] Early on in their new positions, leaders need skills training, such as in performance improvement and conflict resolution. They also need mentors and other support to learn from others, including time to network with others, support for conferences, and support for site visits. In addition to facilitating connections among physicians themselves, there is great opportunity when you provide effective partners for physicians with whom they can work to achieve outcomes, such as nurse coleaders.

When the 20% of physicians are on board, the remaining critical mass of practitioners will learn from their experiences and even add to the initial improvement work. Physician leadership will be viewed as putting physicians at the heart of shaping and running clinical services so as to achieve excellent outcomes for patients and populations, not as a one-off task or project but as a core part of the physician's professional identity.[26]

Make Physicians Partners, Not Customers

Along with aligning priorities with physicians, leaders must work to shift physicians' perspective on their role in the organization. As previously noted, many hospital leaders believe that physicians are important customers who make care decisions while the organization leadership runs the finances and facilities. Likewise, physicians often believe they must have complete autonomy for everything and take personal responsibility only for the patients they take care of directly.

These viewpoints are not productive for the organization, physicians, or patients. To provide the most effective and safe care, patients, families, and the community should be the only customers of a health care organization, and physicians should be partners in providing care to them.

Organizational leadership must set expectations for this perspective shift and support those expectations by consistent practice. Leaders should work with physicians who understand that the patient is the only customer and want to build systems together to support patient needs. Most physicians went into medicine because they want to provide care for people and thus should support the idea of putting the patient at the center of the work.

Unfortunately, some physicians may not like this perspective shift, and in those cases leaders must respond consistently. Physicians who are not willing to give up autonomy for a systematic approach should be encouraged to practice elsewhere. Consider the following scenario:

At the quarterly meeting of the Board Quality Committee, a community board member asks about the medical record delinquency data. The Medical Director says "Yes, we have one or two serial offenders, but one of them is our key trauma surgeon. His op notes and D/C summaries are always months behind. But if we suspended his privileges, as called for in the bylaws, our trauma program would pretty much shut down."

In your institution, what would happen next? Ideally, the trauma surgeon should be held accountable to the same standards as everyone else and disciplined accordingly if he is not willing to change his behavior. If you do not have a single standard—one set of rules—it is very hard to preserve accountability and have a culture that is perceived as fair. This is a key point.

Engage Nurses and Other Clinicians

Organizations that are going to be successful need to invest in a skilled, stable nursing workforce. A simple measure of stability is your organization's annual rate of voluntary nursing turnover. Ideally, it should be close to zero, such as the 0.4% rate at the Dana-Farber Cancer Institute in Boston.[31] With a United States national average at around 10%, where is your organization?[32]

When one skilled nurse leaves an organization, not only does it cost as much as $88,000 to replace him or her, according to one report,[33] but new hires are often not experienced enough to provide the same level of safe, reliable care. Putting brand new graduates in ICUs, operating rooms, and other high-acuity areas without a few years to develop expertise can be more than costly—it can be dangerous. Having skilled people at the bedside is essential for safe care and organizational health.

What are the keys to a healthy nursing environment?

• Creating and maintaining an environment that requires and attracts better-educated nurses, acknowledges their value, and supports ongoing learning

• Eliminating occupational injuries to nurses (and all staff) as a palpable way of communicating that these profes-sionals are an invaluable resource and cannot provide the best possible care to patients when they themselves are not at their best

• Creating a staff professional development program and a nursing leadership structure that provides skilled nurse leaders and managers to support frontline nurses

• Fostering collegial nurse-physician relationships and having zero tolerance for destructive behaviors (such as lack of civility, disrespect, and disruption) both among nurses and between nurses and physicians[34]

• Committing to programs that help build organizational excellence in nursing, such as the American Association of Critical Care Nurses Healthy Work Environments Standard and the American Nurses Credentialing Center (ANCC) Magnet Recognition Program

All of these responsibilities fall directly within the purview of senior leaders.

HIRE FOR WHAT YOU ASPIRE TO BECOME

Although the military has proven through processes such as boot camp that it is possible to rapidly shape another's attitudes and behaviors in alignment with an organization's aspirations, successful companies like Southwest Airlines have found it equally effective to hire the right people in the first place. If your hiring and credentialing process isn't grounded in finding and selecting candidates—physicians, nurses, other clinicians, support staff—who share the organization's core values, possess a desire to serve, have good communication skills, exhibit an eagerness to work in teams, have a commitment to excellence, and communicate an appreciation for feedback, then becoming a reliable and safe organization will take much longer and be much harder than it otherwise should. Although orientation, ongoing training, and daily reinforcement of safety values are essential ingredients in going from good to great in this area, why not give yourself a head start and "get the right people on the bus" to begin with?[35]

INVOLVE BOARD LEADERSHIP IN SAFETY

Physicians and nurses aren't the only groups that are critical to patient safety efforts. Another crucial stakeholder is your organization's board of directors. According to Donald Berwick, then president and CEO of the Institute for Healthcare Improvement (IHI), "Historically, boards have assumed that they are responsible for the fiscal integrity, reputation, and lay management of the hospital, but that responsibility for care lies with the clinical staff, not with the board. For many boards, medical care, itself, is remarkably foreign terrain. Yet, in a time of increasing corporate accountability, consumer voice, and system complexity, this view will no longer suffice, if it ever did. A large share of the accountability for the safety and quality of care rests firmly in the board room. . . . [Cultural changes that support patient safety] require leadership, . . . and in the final analysis, defining the organization's strategic intent and priorities is the responsibility of those who govern the organization."[36]

As Berwick implies, the first step in involving the board in safety and quality efforts is the simple recognition that it is the board's duty in the first place.[37] Better patient outcomes are associated with the following[37]:

• The board spends more than 25% of its time on quality issues.

• The board receives a formal quality performance measurement report.

• There is a high level of interaction between the board and the medical staff on quality strategy.

• The senior executives' compensation is based in part on quality improvement (QI) performance.

• The CEO is identified as the person with the greatest impact on QI.

According to IHI, to assume a major leadership role in improving clinical quality and reducing harm, there are six things all boards should do[36]:

1. Set aims. Set a specific aim to reduce harm this year. Make an explicit, public commitment to measurable quality improvement—such as reducing unnecessary mortality and harm—establishing a clear aim for the facility or system.

2. Get data and hear stories. Select and review progress toward safer care as the first agenda item at every board meeting, grounded in transparency, and putting a "human face" on harm data.

3. Establish and monitor system-level measures. Identify a small group of organizationwide "roll-up" measures of patient safety, such as facilitywide harm or risk-adjusted mortality. Update the measures continually and make them transparent to the entire organization and all of its customers.

4. Change the environment, policies, and culture. Commit to establishing and maintaining an environment

that is respectful, fair, and just for all who experience the pain and loss as a result of avoidable harm and adverse outcomes—the patients, their families, and the staff at the sharp end of error.

5. Learn . . . starting with the board. Develop your capability as a board. Learn about how "best in the world" boards work with executive and physician leaders to reduce harm. Set an expectation for similar levels of education and training for all staff.

6. Establish executive accountability. Oversee the effective execution of a plan to achieve your aim to reduce harm, including executive team accountability for clear quality improvement targets.

The Joint Commission emphasizes the importance of organization leaders' communicating about safety and quality. Through its Leadership standards, The Joint Commission requires organization leaders—including members of the governing body, senior managers, and leaders of the organized medical staff—to communicate with each other on a regular basis with respect to issues of safety and quality.[38]

Obtaining this level of leadership may be challenging, but in its absence, change will be difficult to effect and even more difficult to sustain. Consider beginning the process by engaging each leadership group (the board of directors, CEO, and physician and nursing leaders) in a conversation regarding their level of awareness of the issues, how they view their accountability in this arena, whether they think the organization has the capacity for change, and what explicit actions might be taken to close performance gaps. Consider creating a program in which every new board member and senior leader needs to spend two to four hours shadowing a frontline caregiver. This is a critical perspective they all need. Consider having a patient safety–focused retreat for senior leaders with outside speakers. Often it is easier for external experts to deliver the message of quality and safety and push for significant commitment and improvement.

In an article related to this topic, Frankel, Leonard, and Denham state the following: "Awareness is the first critical dimension. . . . Leaders must be aware of performance gaps before they can commit. . . . Accountability of leaders for closing performance gaps is critical. . . . leaders need to be directly and personally accountable to close the performance gaps. . . . however, [leaders] will fail to close [performance gaps] if their organizations do not have the ability to adopt new practices and technologies. The dimension of ability may be measured as capacity. It includes investment in knowledge, skills, compensated staff time, and 'dark green dollars' of line-item budget allocations."[39(p. 1706)]

To determine if your organization leadership is ready to be effective in achieving safety, initially assess board and senior team performance; and work with the CEO to develop his or her own Leadership Promise using the one provided earlier in this chapter as a guide. Finally, evaluate whether you have respected physicians and other leaders who are or are willing to act as champions of change. They must be willing to publicly commit their support among their peers and express the importance of various efforts. They must also be willing to openly deal with resistance from their colleagues in a constructive manner and insist on a professional culture that won't tolerate nonprofessional behavior. Clear board and CEO support and commitment on these last two points is critically important for success.

In summary, committed, capable, and engaged leadership is essential to systematically improving care and building a culture that makes improvement sustainable.

REFERENCES

1. National Quality Forum (NQF). *Safe Practices for Better Healthcare—2010 Update: A Consensus Report.* Washington, DC: NQF, 2010. Accessed Oct 29, 2012. http://www.qualityforum.org/WorkArea/linkit.aspx?LinkIdentifier=id&ItemID=25689.
2. Botwinick L, Bisognano M, Haraden C. *Leadership Guide to Patient Safety.* IHI Innovation Series white paper. Cambridge, MA: Institute for Healthcare Improvement, 2006. Accessed Oct 29, 2012. http://www.ihi.org/knowledge/Pages/IHIWhitePapers/LeadershipGuidetoPatientSafetyWhitePaper.aspx.
3. Bennis WG, Thomas RJ. *Leading for a Lifetime: How Defining Moments Shape Leaders of Today and Tomorrow.* Boston: Harvard Business School Press, 2007.
4. Rose J, et al. A leadership framework for culture change in health care. *Jt Comm J Qual Patient Saf.* 2006;32(8):433–442.
5. Weick KE, Sutcliffe KM. *Managing the Unexpected: Assuring High Performance in an Age of Complexity.* San Francisco: Jossey-Bass, 2001.
6. Connor M, et al. Creating a fair and just culture: One institution's path toward organizational change. *Jt Comm J Qual Patient Saf.* 2007;33(10):617–624.
7. Nunes J, McFerran S. The perinatal patient safety project: New can be great! *Perm J.* 2005;9(1):25–27.
8. Leonard M, Graham S, Bonacum D. The human factor: The critical importance of effective teamwork and communication in providing safe care. *Qual Saf Health Care.* 2004;13 Suppl 1:i85–90.
9. Pryor DB, et al. The clinical transformation of Ascension Health: Eliminating all preventable injuries and death. *Jt Comm J Qual Patient Saf.* 2006;32(6):299–308.
10. Berwick DM, et al. The 100,000 Lives Campaign: Setting a goal and a deadline for improving health care quality *JAMA.* 2006 Jan 18;295(3):324–327.
11. Institute for Healthcare Improvement. 5 Million Lives Campaign: Overview. Accessed Oct 29, 2012. http://www.ihi.org/offerings/Initiatives/PastStrategicInitiatives/5MillionLivesCampaign/Pages/default.aspx.
12. Frankel A, et al. Patient Safety Leadership WalkRounds™ at Partners Healthcare: Learning from implementation. *Jt Comm J Qual Patient Saf.* 2005;31(8):423–437.
13. Mazzocco K, et al. Surgical team behaviors and patient outcomes. *Am J Surg.* 2009;197(5):678–685.
14. Hudson DW, et al. A safety culture primer for the critical care clinician: The role of culture in patient safety and quality improvement. *Contemporary Critical Care.* 2009;7(5):1–11.
15. Vigorito MC, et al. Improving safety culture results in Rhode Island ICUs: Lessons learned from the development of action-oriented plans. *Jt Comm J Qual Patient Saf.* 2011;37(11):509–514.
16. Langley GL, et al. *The Improvement Guide: A Practical Approach to Enhancing Organizational Performance,* 2nd ed. San Francisco: Jossey-Bass; 2009.
17. Frankel A, Haraden C. Shuttling toward a safety culture: Healthcare can learn from probe panel's findings on the *Columbia* disaster. *Mod Healthc.* 2004;5;34(1):21.
18. Roberts KH, Bea RG. Must accidents happen: Lessons from high reliability organizations. *Academy of Management Executive.* 2001;15(3):70–79.
19. Reason J. *Managing the Risks of Organizational Accidents.* Burlington, VT: Ashgate, 1997.
20. Outcome Engenuity. The Just Culture Community. Accessed Oct 29, 2012. http://www.justculture.org.
21. University of Pittsburgh Medical Center: Condition Help. Accessed Oct 29, 2012. http://www.upmc.com/about/why-upmc/quality/excellence-in-patient-care/Pages/condition-h.aspx.
22. Institute for Patient- and Family-Centered Care. Home page. Accessed Oct 29, 2012. http://www.ipfcc.org.
23. Dana-Farber Cancer Institute. Establishing Patient- and Family-Centered Care. Accessed Oct 29, 2012. http://www.dana-farber.org/Pediatric-Care/New-Patient-Guide/Patient-and-Family-Advisory-Council/Establishing-Patient-and-Family-Centered-Care.aspx.
24. Beth Israel Deaconess Medical Center: Chat with Paul Levy. Accessed Nov 10, 2008; no longer available online.
25. Snell AJ, Briscoe D, Dickson G. From the inside out: The engagement of physicians as leaders in health care settings. *Qual Health Res.* 2011;21(7):952–967.
26. Mountford J, Webb C. *Clinical Leadership: Unlocking High Performance in Healthcare.* London: McKinsey & Company, Aug 2008. Accessed Oct 29, 2012. http://www.knowledge.scot.nhs.uk/media/CLT/ResourceUploads/22024/200908%20Clinical%20Leadership%20doc%20by%20MckinseyAug08.pdf.
27. Reinertsen Group. Achieving Clinical Integration with Highly Engaged Physicians. Gosfield A, Reinertsen J. 2010. Accessed Oct 29, 2012. http://www.reinertsengroup.com/publications/documents/True%20Clinical%20Integration%20Gosfield%20Reinertsen%202010.pdf.
28. Lee TH. Turning doctors into leaders. *Harv Bus Rev.* 2010;88(4):50–58.
29. NHS Institute for Innovation and Improvement and Academy of Medical Royal Colleges: *Medical Leadership Competency Framework: Enhancing Engagement in Medical Leadership,* 3rd ed. Coventry, UK: NHS Institute for Innovation and Improvement and Academy of Medical Royal Colleges, Jul 2010. Accessed Oct 29, 2012. http://www.institute.nhs.uk/images/documents/Medical%20Leadership%20Competency%20Framework%203rd%20ed.pdf.
30. Healthcare Leadership Alliance. Introducing the HLA Competency Directory, Version 2.0. 2010. Accessed Oct 29, 2012. http://www.healthcareleadershipalliance.org.
31. Hayes C, et al. Retaining oncology nurses: Strategies for today's nurse leaders. *Oncol Nurs Forum.* 2005;32(6):1087–1090. Accessed Oct 29,

2012. http://ons.metapress.com/content/t9825427n6941880/
?p=ac2ad63040ce4de49fd884cad022053d&pi=3.

32. DeFontes J, Surbida S. Preoperative safety briefing project. *Perm J.*
2004;8(2):21–27. Accessed Oct 29, 2012. http://xnet.kp.org/
permanentejournal/spring04/awardwin.pdf.

33. Jones CB. Revisiting nurse turnover costs: Adjusting for inflation. *J Nurs
Adm.* 2008;38(1):11–18.

34. Institute of Medicine. *To Err Is Human: Building a Better Health System.*
Washington, DC: National Academy Press, 2000.

35. Collins J. *Good to Great: Why Some Companies Make the Leap . . . and
Others Don't.* New York City: HarperBusiness/HarperCollins, 2001.

36. Institute for Healthcare Improvement: The Power of Having the Board
on Board. (Updated: Aug 1, 2011.) Accessed Oct 28, 2012.
http://www.ihi.org/knowledge/Pages/ImprovementStories/
ThePowerofHavingtheBoardonBoard.aspx.

37. Vaughn T, et al. Engagement of leadership in quality improvement
initiatives: Executive quality improvement survey results. *J Patient Saf.*
2006;2(1):2–9. Accessed Oct 29, 2012. http://www.cha.com/pdfs/
Quality/Tools%20and%20Resources/
vaughnetalengagementofleadershipinqiinitiatives_jpatsafetymar06.pdf.

38. The Joint Commission. *2012 Comprehensive Accreditation Manual for
Hospitals: The Official Handbook.* Oak Brook, IL: Joint Commission
Resources, 2011.

39. Frankel AS, Leonard MW, Denham CR. Fair and just culture, team
behavior, and leadership engagement: The tools to achieve high reliability.
Health Serv Res. 2006;41(4 Pt 2):1690–1709.

Chapter Two

ASSESSING AND IMPROVING SAFETY CULTURE

Natasha Scott, MSc; Allan Frankel, MD; Michael Leonard, MD

In this chapter, we address the topic of safety culture—explaining why it is important and describing leadership's critical role in building and sustaining it. We also discuss how to measure safety culture and offer practical mechanisms to link safety culture insights to action.

WHAT IS SAFETY CULTURE?

Edgar Schein has systematically studied culture for more than five decades. In Schein's model of culture, there are artifacts, espoused values, and underlying basic assumptions.[1]

Artifacts

Artifacts are the visible pieces of culture, the observable behaviors and work processes you see and hear as you walk through a clinical unit. The next time you are working in or visiting a clinical unit, look around for the stated values posted on the wall. Are there visible and transparent communication venues that highlight unit learning and possible improvement opportunities? How are caregivers interacting with one another? For example, do you see surgeons using the back stairways to come onto the unit to see their patients and leave the same way without stopping by the nursing station to spend a few minutes discussing the plan of care with the nurses? All these observed pieces of culture can be considered artifacts.

Espoused Values

Espoused values are the values that everyone in the unit declares they hold and support, and they reflect the *desired* behavior of caregivers. A common example of an espoused value is "we are committed to working together to deliver optimal care for every patient through collaboration and effective communication." This espoused value reflects the

desired behavior of caregivers to effectively collaborate and communicate with one another. If we went to a clinical unit and talked to caregivers from physicians to housekeepers, we would hear the espoused values, describing how they see their work and what they believe is important.

Espoused values may or may not be consistent with *observed* behavior or artifacts. For example, on one clinical unit where the above espoused value was present, a desired behavior associated with the espoused value was for nurses to turn patients from one side to the other every 60 minutes to prevent pressure ulcers. However, what was observed on this unit was that the nurses tended to "dump work on each other," so patients would not get turned reliably, and dressing changes waited until the next shift.

Underlying Basic Assumptions

Underlying basic assumptions represent the assumptions that all caregivers working on a unit make about how to deliver patient care. These basic assumptions determine the observable behaviors or artifacts. These assumptions are so ingrained in the unit that if someone suggests an alternative way of doing things, this person would be immediately dismissed and thought of as "crazy." Changing these basic assumptions is a difficult process because it necessitates challenging people's reality.

When people refer to culture change as a long, slow process that does not happen overnight, they are often specifically referring to changing the underlying basic assumptions of a unit or organization. A common basic assumption that has been held for many decades in health care is that physicians know what is best for a patient. In units where this basic assumption is present, it would be considered highly unusual for a nurse to know more about what the patient needs than a physician, and it would be inconceivable for a nurse or any other caregiver to ever question anything a physician says or does.

Defining Safety Culture

Taken together, the artifacts, espoused values, and underlying basic assumptions indicate the type of culture an organization has. Espoused values and artifacts, as concrete aspects of culture, can be relatively easily understood and assessed, while it is more challenging to uncover the underlying basic assumptions about how patient care is delivered. Artifacts and espoused values are also referred to as the *safety climate*.[2] The more concordant a culture is regarding the artifacts, espoused values, and underlying basic assumptions present, the healthier it is. A culture can be considered "safe" when the artifacts, espoused values, and underlying basic assumptions all support and reinforce that patient safety is a top priority throughout the organization.

If espoused values are greatly at odds with the observed behaviors and underlying basic assumptions, then the culture is an unsafe one for everyone.

A more practical description of safety culture within health care is as follows:

- Optimal, safe care is everyone's overarching, non-negotiable goal.
- No one is ever hesitant to voice a concern about a patient because it is psychologically safe to do so.
- There is a simple, clear model of accountability that clearly differentiates "unsafe" individuals from competent, conscientious individuals who "fall victim to" system errors. People need to know they're safe before they're going to be comfortable talking about errors, near misses, and system failures.
- There is a continual focus on identifying and mitigating sources of risks and hazards
- When individuals do voice concerns, they know they will be treated with respect, and leadership will address their concerns and take action.
- After leaders have taken action or looked into the matter, they will close the loop and provide feedback to the person who raised the concern.

Psychological Safety Is a Critical Element

One essential element of safety culture is psychological safety, which has been extensively studied by Edmondson and Schein.[3,4] While Chapter 6 takes a detailed look at this topic, here we aim to put the concept in context. Think of your own experience in your training and current clinical work. How often are individual team members invited to speak up, and what is their experience when they do? If they are treated with respect, and their concerns are acted upon, they are far more likely to speak up in the future. That's psychological safety. If they are not treated respectfully, they are far less likely to voice a future concern, which creates risk. You know the people you are always comfortable going to if you have a question or a problem, because they will not only help you but also treat you with respect. The converse is that the people you're hesitant to approach because it wasn't too much fun the last time you approached them. This hesitation is dangerous in a health care setting because it can lead to clinicians hesitating to voice concerns about a patient.

Lack of psychological safety creates unacceptable risk for both patients and caregivers. Sadly, there are many studies that show caregivers who failed to speak up while observing mistakes being made or patients deteriorating because it didn't feel safe for them to speak up.[5-7] Patients entrust their lives to us every day; leaders have a fundamental obligation to support a safety culture in which it is never acceptable to be concerned about a patient and not speak up.

LINKING CULTURE AND LEADERSHIP

Leadership plays an important role in establishing and maintaining safety culture. Krause's extensive work in industrial safety demonstrates that the safest organizations, that also tend to be operationally quite efficient, have two basic qualities: clearly defined behaviors that apply to everyone and a continual focus on improving organizational culture.[8]

Processes that systematically connect leadership to the activities and concerns of frontline caregivers have great value. It is quite difficult, if not impossible, to drive a safety culture in the absence of such mechanisms. In many health care systems today, caregivers have little confidence that information they provide will be acted on and/or they will receive feedback from leadership. We have frequently heard staff comment in effect, "Ideas and concerns just go off into a black hole and we never hear back, so we got tired of telling them—if they don't care, why should we?"

To support, foster, and encourage safety culture, it can be helpful to focus on one or two aspects first, as Tucker and Singer have shown; organizations were far better off asking frontline staff about one or two things that were important to them, acting on them, and providing feedback.[9] This reinforces the dynamic that "leadership is here to help us, we go to them, they listen to us, they fix it if they can, and they come back and tell us." Conversely, when leaders solicited multiple suggestions for improvement and did not provide feedback as to what was learned and what they did, the culture went backward.

One effective way to encourage a systematic flow of information between caregivers at the bedside and leadership is Leadership WalkRounds. As discussed in detail in Chapter 5, WalkRounds provides an infrastructure for not only regularly engaging leaders and frontline caregivers in a dialogue as to how to provide safer care and fix defects but also handling information so it is analyzed and acted on, and feedback is provided to 100% of the people who provide information. This can support the creation and maintenance of a safety culture. Although WalkRounds is not a casual process, it is scripted to seem natural and casual in the questions asked and how it is managed.[10]

WHY IS SAFETY CULTURE IMPORTANT?

There is progressively more evidence that links safety culture to better patient care, improved patient outcomes, and a safer work environment. Consider, for example, the following studies:

• Knaus et al., in a multicenter ICU study, looked at the relationship of safety culture to patient outcomes. Patients in units with a higher safety culture had significantly better (risk-adjusted) outcomes.[11]

• In the Michigan Keystone project in which ICUs systematically implemented a central line bundle to reduce infections, the overall result was an impressive 70% reduction in infection rates. It is projected that the ICUs saved 1,200 lives as well as approximately 200 million dollars. Before the intervention, safety culture was measured in each of the 103 ICUs as a baseline. After the intervention, researchers looked to see if there was a correlation between inherent ICU culture and the ability to achieve five months or more with zero infections. Looking across the safety culture distribution, 44% of the upper one third of units (those with a higher safety culture) achieved the goal, whereas only 21% of the lower one third of units (those with a lower safety culture) achieved the goal.[12]

• Hansen and his colleagues, who examined 30-day readmission rates for patients with congestive heart failure and coronary artery disease, found that as positive perceptions of safety climate increased, readmission rates fell. Nurses' perceptions were more accurate in assessing risk in congestive heart failure, while physicians' perceptions were more predictive in coronary artery disease.[13]

• Curry et al. found that the highest-performing hospitals with respect to acute coronary syndromes had not only systematic processes but also a central focus on organizational culture.[14]

• In a surgical safety initiative across 74 hospitals in the Veterans Health Administration, Neily et al. reported that hospitals that focused on structured communication and teamwork, process improvement, and learning saw an 18% reduction in mortality, significant improvement in surgical care measures, more efficient use of operating rooms, and significant improvements in safety culture.[15]

• A critical care collaborative in Rhode Island found significant increases in safety culture scores and improved clinical outcomes after adopting a structured debriefing process for its safety culture data.[16,17]

These studies together suggest that being able to accurately measure and reflect the perceptions of team members at a unit level and reach common agreement as to how the team will communicate and treat each other has significant implications for the quality of care delivered and the quality of work life for the people delivering care.

ASSESSING SAFETY CULTURE

Safety culture is not something that can be easily seen or observed. Organizations must assess safety culture by using a multifaceted approach, much like diagnosing a patient. Most often when a patient arrives at a health care organization, the status of his or her health is not immediately known just by looking at him or her. A physician has to perform a series of examinations and tests (such as blood pressure, heart rate, blood work, and so forth) to properly diagnose the patient's symptoms and get a comprehensive understanding of his or her overall health. The same can be said for the culture of an organization. You cannot get a complete understanding of the health of the culture just by looking at the organization or a specific clinical area without conducting a series of diagnostic tests and exams. Conducting safety culture assessments gives you the data and information required to make an accurate diagnosis of the overall health of the culture.

The data from safety culture assessments provide information about where there are opportunities for patient safety improvement and help you develop systematic strategies to achieve that improvement. Specifically, safety culture assessments do the following:

• Help leaders prioritize which clinical areas across a hospital require the most support in quality and safety improvement

• Identify specific culture dimensions on which to focus patient safety improvement efforts (for example, improvement in teamwork and communication, leadership, psychological safety)

• Provide a method of determining if patient safety improvement initiatives are successful by using a pre- and postintervention assessment approach

• Help normalize open discussion of cultural issues that affect patient safety, which quickens the process of getting at the root of patient safety issues and how to fix them

One can think of individuals conducting culture assessments as "cultural doctors." In fact, the characteristics of a good cultural doctor are the same as a good medical doctor. Best practices for both include the following:

1. Having a high level of knowledge, expertise, and competence in the area

2. Using valid tools and assessment methods to make a diagnosis

3. Performing a comprehensive assessment before making any conclusions

Types of Safety Culture Assessments

Safety culture assessments can be done at either the organizational level (across a hospital, for example) or the unit level (in a specific clinical area). Culture in health care tends to be local, meaning that there is often significant variation in culture between units or departments. It is very possible to have two units (for example, surgical and ICU units) that are very close in proximity—15 feet apart from one another— with two completely different cultures. One unit could have a collegial atmosphere in which everyone treats one another with respect regardless of position and everyone feels comfortable speaking up. Conversely, the other unit could have a negative atmosphere in which individuals are ridiculed if they voice a concern about a patient.

Campbell et al. reported a study in which 2,163 physicians and nurses associated with specific clinical units completed a safety culture survey. Ratings of various safety climate domains differed markedly across the 57 units, the percentage of respondents reporting a safety grade of "excellent," for example, ranged from 0% to 50%. Even within the six unit types, substantial variation across individual units was evident.[18]

Unit-level safety culture assessments are the best way to capture this variation. Results from such assessments can be used to develop tailored improvement plans for each unit.

The Process of Safety Culture Assessment

Regardless of whether you chose to conduct an organizational or unit-level culture assessment, the process is similar. Fleming developed a useful how-to guide for conducting safety culture assessments, which breaks the process down into 10 basic steps.[19] These steps are summarized in Sidebar 2-1 on page 17.

SAFETY CULTURE ASSESSMENT TOOLS

Surveys are the most frequently used safety culture assessment tool in health care (*see* Sidebar 2-2 on page 17 for some alternative methods of safety culture assessment). There are a number of benefits to using surveys when assessing patient safety culture. First, the survey method provides a standardized assessment because everyone completing a survey answers the same questions, using the same response options, typically ranging from strongly disagree to strongly agree. Second, surveys can be comprehensive as they can be administered to everyone within the health care organization. Third, surveys are efficient in terms of the time it takes to complete the typical patient safety culture survey (usually around 10–20 minutes). Finally, a nice feature of safety culture surveys is the ability to benchmark survey results and make comparisons across units or hospitals. Given the extensive use of safety culture surveys in health care, a number of best practices have been identified (*see* Sidebar 2-3 on page 18).

Administering a safety culture survey is a time- and resource-intensive process, and it is easy to get overwhelmed by the amount of work involved. Fortunately, there are a number of organizations that specialize in administering safety culture surveys. These companies have standard processes to ensure that survey administration runs

Sidebar 2-1. 10 Steps to Conducting a Safety Culture Assessment

1. **Acquire expertise.** Ensure that you have the right expertise and competence to conduct a safety culture assessment; identifying your "cultural doctors" will get you off to a good start.

2. **Select an appropriate assessment instrument.** Identify an instrument that meets your needs (organizational vs. unit-level assessment) and is valid.

3. **Obtain informed leadership support.** Senior leadership support often determines the success or failure of safety culture assessments. Senior leaders need to understand what is involved in the assessment process and have a clear understanding of their responsibilities. Conducting a leadership briefing at the beginning of this process can help build leadership support.

4. **Involve frontline staff.** Staff involvement is a key characteristic of a positive safety culture. Involve frontline staff to build interest and engagement in both the assessment and in the patient safety improvement initiatives that follow. One way of involving frontline staff is by having staff champions who promote the process.

5. **Conduct the assessment.** It is now time to implement!

6. **Analyze and interpret data.** Understand what the results of the assessment mean.

7. **Communicate the results.** You have told everyone you are doing a safety culture assessment, many have directly participated in the assessment itself, now it is time to close the loop with these individuals. Results of the safety culture assessment should be widely distributed. Conduct debriefing sessions with both leadership and frontline staff (separately).

8. **Develop an action plan.** Identify practical solutions that can be implemented to make a real difference in patient safety. Solutions should be developed in partnership with frontline staff.

9. **Implement the action plan.** It is once again time to implement. This step should closely follow steps 5–8 while there is still momentum from the assessment itself. The longer you wait to implement an action plan, the harder it is to connect it to the assessment.

10. **Track improvement.** The primary goal of conducting a safety culture assessment is to identify areas for improvement. The initial assessment can serve as a baseline measure. Completing follow-up assessments will allow you to determine if changes have occurred.

Source: Adapted from Fleming M. Patient safety culture measurement and improvement: A "how-to" guide. *Health Q.* 2005;8 Spec No:14–19. Accessed Oct 30, 2012. http://www.longwoods.com/content/17656.

Sidebar 2-2. Other Safety Culture Assessment Methods

Focus Groups

Focus groups are an alternative to safety culture surveys. Similar to a survey approach, the purpose of the focus group is to collect information regarding frontline staff's perceptions of the culture. Focus groups work best when there is a facilitator guiding the discussion and taking notes (or recording the session) and when there are 6–12 participants of the same seniority. The number of focus groups is dependent on the size of the organization. It has been suggested that focus groups should sample a minimum of 10%–20% of employees.[1]

Having a skilled facilitator is key. Facilitators should be perceived as neutral by the participants so they feel comfortable speaking up. Facilitators should also be well-trained in how to structure the discussion in order to get the most information from participants, while at the same time not letting the focus group experience turn into a venting session.[1]

Patient Safety Culture Audits

Audit tools assess organization-level indicators of patient safety culture and are useful for identifying which patient safety practices the organization is doing well, which practices need to be improved, and which important patient safety practices the organization is not currently doing at all.[2] A team of senior administrative leaders, clinical leaders, and frontline staff should complete patient safety culture audit tools. There are several instruments currently available, including one developed by Fleming and Wentzell,[2] and another in use at the University of Manchester.[3]

References
1. International Atomic Energy Agency (IAEA). *Self-Assessment of Safety Culture in Nuclear Installations: Highlights and Good Practices.* Technical Document No. 1321. Vienna: IAEA, 2002.
2. VHA, Inc. Strategies for Leadership: An Organizational Approach to Patient Safety. Irving, TX, 2000. Accessed Jul 19, 2012. http://www.aha.org/content/00-10/VHAtool.pdf.
3. Fleming M, Wentzell N. Patient safety culture improvement tool: Development and guidelines for use. *Healthcare Q.* 2008;11 (3 Spec No.) 10–15. Accessed Oct 30, 2012. http://www.longwoods.com/content/19604.
4. University of Manchester. Manchester Patient Safety Assessment Framework. Accessed Oct 30, 2012. http://www.pharmacy.manchester.ac.uk/cip/resources/MaPSafPart1.pdf.

smoothly, and they have standard reporting mechanisms, which typically means a quick turnaround of survey results. On the other hand, if you have the resources and the desire to administer the survey yourself, you may have more control over the survey and survey process.

1. What Survey Should We Use?

During the past decade, a number of patient safety culture surveys have been developed.[20–23] In choosing a survey, it is important to consider your specific organizational context and select a survey that meets your organization's needs. For example, a survey should measure the topics that are of most interest to you and be versatile enough to use across the different areas and caregivers you wish to assess. Figure 2-1 on page 20 describes the two most popular safety culture surveys in health care, the Safety Attitudes Questionnaire (SAQ)[20] and the Hospital Survey on Patient Safety Culture (HSOPS).[24]

Sidebar 2-3. Safety Culture Survey Best Practices

- Surveys should be administered across the hospital or health care system.
- Use a census approach to survey administration in which all individuals in the organization are invited to complete the survey.
- Ensure that survey responses are anonymous and confidential; this will encourage staff to respond honestly.
- Mapping survey responses to a particular unit is important for assessing unit-level culture (this can be done without identifying individual responses).
- Use a validated survey; a survey should be reliable (performance of survey items should be consistent over time), accurately and thoroughly measure the constructs or topics it is designed to measure, and be predictive of clinical and operational outcomes (such as bloodstream infection rates, turnover.
- Develop communication materials to promote the survey. Before the survey is administered, staff members should be informed of the purpose of the survey, why it's important for them to complete it, and any logistical information (such as the length of time they have to complete the survey, how they will be receiving the survey, and so on). Communication materials should be brief and concise. Use a variety of communication forums (for example, e-mail, newsletters, websites, announcements at staff meetings) to ensure that the message is being received.

Source: Natasha Scott, Pascal Metrics, Inc. Used with permission.

---

2. What Type of Survey Modality Should We Use?

There are several ways to administer a survey. The most common modalities are paper and electronic. Paper surveys can be "group administered." For example, it is common practice to ask individuals to complete a survey during the first or last 15 minutes of a staff meeting. It is also common to schedule specific sessions during working hours for staff to complete the survey. This is more easily done with paper surveys than electronic surveys simply because of a lack of computer resources. Electronic surveys on the other hand can be easier to administer and manage as they allow for sending mass e-mail survey invites, tracking response rates in real-time, and sending e-mail reminders.

3. What Are We Going to Do to Help Ensure a High Survey Response Rate?

A high response rate is critical for the success of a safety culture survey. In the safety culture work that we do across several hundred hospitals, the average response rate is between 75% and 85%. We set a minimum threshold at 60%. The reason for this is to ensure statistically valid data and maintain confidence that repeat surveys will be measuring the same population of respondents. Low response rates make it harder to interpret the results and develop improvement plans because you cannot be sure the results are accurate and generalizable across the unit. Considering how to increase response rates before you start survey administration will help to avoid the panic that often follows from seeing low response rates for the first time. *See* Sidebar 2-4 on page 19 for some tips on how to improve response rates.

LINKING SAFETY CULTURE ASSESSMENT TO IMPROVEMENT

High-quality safety culture data are powerful for engaging senior leaders and frontline staff to focus on and drive improvement. Analysis of the data provides a broad view of cultural themes across the organization and also more granular perspectives about caregiver perceptions at a unit level. Data analysis will help delineate strengths that can be leveraged, such as perceptions of teamwork or organizational commitment to safe care, and also areas of weakness that exist across the organization that can be targeted as strategic initiatives.

Safety culture really "lives" at a unit level, as stated earlier, with most organizations, in our experience, averaging

Sidebar 2-4. Tips for Achieving a High Response Rate

The Agency for Healthcare Research and Quality (AHRQ) has provided information on how to increase survey response rates. Following are a few of the tips offered.

Get leadership involved. Get leaders at all levels in the organization to sponsor and promote the survey.

Market the survey. Develop a promotional campaign that includes multiple methods of communication (for example, e-mails, newsletters, bulletin boards, websites).

Create friendly competition. Throughout the data collection phase, distribute unit and facility response rates so each unit/facility can compare how it is doing against other units/facilities.

Provide incentives. Provide prize incentives for units (such as a free lunch for the unit achieving the highest response rate) and/or individual lottery draws, including movie tickets, a few hours of paid leave, and so forth.

A note of caution when using incentives: External incentives, such as prizes, can distract from the real purpose of the survey (understanding the safety culture of the unit so patient safety can be improved). Such incentives may lead to individuals halfheartedly completing the survey just to get their name entered into a draw, instead of providing thoughtful responses. To avoid this problem, ensure that both the importance of the survey and the incentives are given equal focus.

Source: Agency for Healthcare Research and Quality. Surveys on Patient Safety Culture: Establishing Data Collection Procedures: Maximize Your Response Rate. Accessed Oct 30, 2012. http://www.ahrq.gov/qual/patientsafetyculture/hospcult5.htm.

on the unit. For example, in an operating room where 85% of the surgeons think that nursing input is well received, and only 20% of the nurses think so, there is significant dysfunction and potential risk and an opportunity for improvement. The power of high-quality safety culture data is that they are personal and offer profound insight as to what it really feels like to be delivering care within a clinical setting. High response rates with individual caregiver perceptions quickly deals with data validity and allows for respectful, but straightforward, conversations.

Looking at strong units provides insight into best practices that can be spread, or the potential to partner strong units with ones that are struggling. Observing low-scoring units that are involved in higher-risk areas of care, such as obstetrics, surgery, critical care, or emergency care, and correlating lows scores with adverse events, quality metrics, and episodes of patient harm can help organizations be strategic on where to focus safety efforts. It is far more productive to focus on a few clinical areas of real opportunity where there can be sustained attention and measurable improvement than go too broadly into a "spray and pray" approach across the health system that will not be sustainable and runs the risk of being perceived as another "flavor of the month" improvement exercise.

The process of linking safety culture assessment to measurable activities that drive improvement requires a robust and systematic process of debriefing safety culture results. The primary rule of debriefing, which cannot be violated, is that the whole intent of the process is to find opportunity and drive improvement. Creating an environment of psychological safety is essential for debriefing to be successful. The dialogue can never be judgmental or engage in blame. Anchoring with the premise that "we're all here to provide optimal, safe care for every patient, and create an environment that keeps us safe" is a good way to start. Having high-quality safety culture data that reflect the strengths and weaknesses of the unit-level culture provides personal context of strengths that can be leveraged.

Sexton et al. describe a unit-level debriefing process in which a multidisciplinary team examines its safety culture results—in terms of both strengths and weaknesses—and focuses on one area that is important to the people in the unit, noting why it is important and committing to measurable action.[25] As previously mentioned, this process, when applied in the Rhode Island ICU Collaborative, resulted in

a five-to-sixfold variation across units, so that drilling down cultural data and looking at caregiver perceptions at a unit level are essential. Examination will most likely show very strong units with high perceptions of teamwork and safety climate, and units that are weak in one or both areas.

The hallmark of a healthy safety culture in a given unit is that the relative perceptions of individuals working in the unit, including housekeepers, unit secretaries, technicians, nurses, physicians, and managers, are concordant on the topic of teamwork and safety. In other words, in a healthy safety culture, there is a "good movie and everyone is in the same one." In dysfunctional units, there are often different perceptions of what it feels like to deliver care and interact broad improvements in safety culture and clinical improvement regarding bloodstream infections and ventilator-associated pneumonia in units that used debriefing and little to no change in the ICUs that did not.

Combining high-quality safety culture measurement with debriefing and commitment to actionable, measurable improvement is currently seen by multiple large health care systems as an important driver of improvement. Allan Frankel's Team-Based Engagement Model (TEM) co-developed with the Mayo Clinic, provides a comprehensive mechanism for assessing unit-level safety culture, bolstering it with interviews to capture the narrative and gain further context regarding the safety culture. It also embeds team and leadership behaviors such as briefing, critical language, and debriefing and creates a "Learning System" (*see* Chapter 13) to capture insights from the debriefing process and link

these insights to tests of change and measurable improvement cycles. This approach not only creates and builds the capacity of unit-level improvement but also allows unit-level clinicians to work on specific aspects of safety culture and teamwork in a sustainable manner.

CONCLUSION

Safety culture is the mortar that holds the bricks together; it is foundational to all patient safety work. Assessing an organization's safety culture is a critical step in the patient safety journey. Gaining leadership support, using a valid and reliable tool, effectively conducting the survey, and linking results to measurable improvement activities in a way that engages both leadership and frontline staff are essential to laying the foundation for improvement work and ultimately enhancing the care you provide to patients.

Figure 2-1. A Brief Comparison of Patient Safety Culture Surveys

	Safety Attitudes Questionnaire	Hospital Survey on Patient Safety Culture
Culture Dimensions Measured	1. Teamwork Climate 2. Safety Climate 3. Job Satisfaction 4. Stress Recognition 5. Working Conditions 6. Perceptions of Senior Management 7. Perceptions of Local Management	1. Teamwork Within Units 2. Supervisor/Manager Expectations & Actions Promoting Patient Safety 3. Organizational Learning/Continuous Improvement 4. Management Support for Patient Safety 5. Overall Perceptions of Patient Safety 6. Feedback & Communication About Errors 7. Communication Openness 8. Frequency of Events Reported 9. Teamwork Across Units 10. Staffing 11. Handoffs & Transitions 12. Nonpunitive Response to Errors
Survey Length	34 questions	51 questions
Benchmarking Capabilities	Yes	Yes—Publicly available through AHRQ
Validated	Yes	Yes

Source: Natasha Scott, Pascal Metrics, Inc. Used with permission.

This figure shows a direct comparison between two of the most commonly used patient safety culture surveys. Adapted from the following sources: OpenSafety.org Safety Attitudes Questionnaire, http://www.opensafety.org/opensafetyorg-culture-surveys/; and Agency for Healthcare Research and Quality, Hospital Survey on Patient Safety Culture, http://www.ahrq.gov/qual/patientsafetyculture/hospsurvindex.htm.

REFERENCES

1. Schein EH. *Organizational Culture and Leadership,* 4th ed. San Francisco: Jossey-Bass, 2010.

2. Guldenmund FW. The nature of safety culture: A review of theory and research. *Safety Science.* 2000;34:215–257. Accessed Oct 30, 2012. http://www.tudelft.nl/live/binaries/55e4afad-b4c5-4e33-b60c-68a9c6bcfc3c/doc/safetyscience2000.pdf.

3. Edmondson A. Psychological safety and learning behavior in work teams. Administrative Science Quarterly. 1999;44(2):350–383.

4. Edmondson AC. *Teaming: How Organizations Learn, Innovate, and Compete in the Knowledge Economy.* San Francisco: Jossey-Bass, 2012.

5. Blatt R, et al. A sensemaking lens on reliability. *Journal of Organizational Behavior.* 2006;27(7):897–917.

6. Bognár A, et al. Errors and the burden of errors: Attitudes, perceptions, and the culture of safety in pediatric cardiac surgical teams. *Ann Thorac Surg.* 2008;85(4):1374–1381.

7. Institute for Safe Medication Practices. Medication Safety Alert! Intimidation: Practitioners speak up about this unresolved problem (Part I). Mar 11, 2004. Accessed Oct 30, 2012. http://www.ismp.org/Newsletters/acutecare/articles/20040311_2.asp.

8. Krause TR. *Leading with Safety.* Hoboken, NJ: Wiley, 2005.

9. Tucker AL, Singer SJ. Determinants of successful frontline process improvement: Action versus analysis (Harvard Business School working paper). Cambridge, MA, 2011. Accessed Oct 30, 2012. http://www.hbs.edu/research/pdf/10-047.pdf.

10. Frankel A, et al. Patient Safety Leadership WalkRounds™ at Partners Healthcare: Learning from implementation. *Jt Comm J Qual Patient Saf.* 2005;31(8):423–437.

11. Knaus WA, et al. An evaluation of outcome from intensive care in major medical centers. *Ann Intern Med.* 1986;104(3):410–418.

12. Hudson DW, et al. A safety culture primer for the critical care clinician: The role of culture in patient safety and quality improvement. *Contemporary Critical Care.* 2009;7(5):1–11.

13. Hansen LO, Williams MV, Singer SJ. Perceptions of hospital safety climate and incidence of readmission. *Health Serv Res.* 2011;46(2):596–616.

14. Curry LA, et al. What distinguishes top-performing hospitals in acute myocardial infarction mortality rates? A qualitative study. *Ann Intern Med.* 2011 Mar 15;154(6):384–390.

15. Neily J, et al. Association between implementation of a medical team training program and surgical mortality. *JAMA.* 2010 Oct 20;304(15):1693–1700.

16. DePalo VA, et al. The Rhode Island ICU collaborative: A model for reducing central line-associated bloodstream infection and ventilator-associated pneumonia statewide. *Qual Saf Health Care.* 2010;19(6):555–561.

17. Chase D. *Rhode Island Quality Institute. A Statewide Partnership to Improve Healthcare Quality.* Commonwealth Fund pub. 1465, vol. 107. New York: Commonwealth Fund, Dec 2010. Accessed Oct 30, 2012. http://www.commonwealthfund.org/-/media/Files/Publications/Case%20Study/2010/Dec/1465_Chase_Rhode_Island_quality_inst_case_study.pdf.

18. Campbell EG, et al. Patient safety climate in hospitals: Act locally on variation across units. *Jt Comm J Qual Patient Saf.* 2010;36(7):319–326.

19. Fleming M. Patient safety culture measurement and improvement: A "how-to" guide. *Healthc Q.* 2005;8 Spec No:14–19. Accessed Oct 30, 2012. http://www.longwoods.com/content/17656.

20. Sexton JB, et al. *Frontline Assessments of Healthcare Culture: Safety Attitudes Questionnaire Norms and Psychometric Properties.* Technical Report No. 04-01. Houston: University of Texas Center of Excellence for Patient Safety Research and Practice, 2004.

21. Sorra J, Nieva V. *Psychometric Analysis of the Hospital Survey on Patient Safety.* Rockville, MD: Westat, under contract to BearingPoint, 2003. Sponsored by the Agency for Healthcare Research and Quality.

22. Singer SJ, et al. The culture of safety: Results from an organization-wide survey in 15 California hospitals. *Qual Saf Health Care.* 2003;12(2):112–118.

23. Ginsburg L, et al. Advancing measurement of patient safety culture. *Health Serv Res.* 2009;44(1):205–224.

24. Agency for Healthcare Research and Quality. Hospital Survey on Patient Safety Culture. (Updated: Jun 2012.) Accessed Oct 30, 2012. http://www.ahrq.gov/qual/patientsafetyculture/hospsurvindex.htm.

25. Sexton JB, et al. A check-up for safety culture in "my patient care area." *Jt Comm J Qual Patient Saf.* 2007;33(11):699–703.

Chapter Three

ACCOUNTABILITY AND THE REALITY OF THE HUMAN CONDITION

Allan Frankel, MD; Frank Federico, RPh; Michael Leonard, MD

When bad things happen a knee-jerk reaction is to look for someone to blame. When something goes wrong, the common tendency is to find out "who did it" rather than "why." Although this approach is understandable in health care because it makes organizations feel as if they have responded to a problem and taken action, the underlying flaw with this approach is that only about 5% of medical harm is caused by incompetent or poorly intended care, and consequently 95% of errors that cause harm involve conscientious, competent individuals who, through a series of system failures, make a mistake that leads to an unintended and sometimes catastrophic result. Consequently, placing blame on an individual does not address the underlying issues that cause harm and does not prevent the harm from happening again.

Consider this example: A dedicated nurse had 15 years of clinical experience as an obstetrical nurse and spent her entire career working on the obstetrical unit of a large Midwestern hospital. She was integral in creating the hospital's infant bereavement program and was a valued asset to the organization.

The obstetrics unit on which the nurse worked did not use float or traveling nurses, so nurses on the unit filled in extra shifts. To encourage nurses to take extra shifts, the hospital gave an award—a trip to a nursing conference—to the nurse who worked the most overtime hours in a given year. One day in July, the nurse worked a double shift of 16 hours. Because the unit was shorthanded, she agreed to work another shift—laid down for 5–6 hours—and resumed patient care.

Of note was that the hospital had recently installed a new bar-coding system, which was working only about two out of three times, and, according to the nurses, had problems reading IV bags, including those that contained antibiotics and local anesthetics.

Also, because the obstetrics (OB) unit did not have anesthesia providers dedicated to OB that were based on the unit, the floor nurses had to request an anesthesiologist to come from the operating room area to the OB unit every time a patient needed an epidural—some 2,000 times a year. To help address the inconvenience of this setup, the hospital had a task force of anesthesia and OB unit providers working on a protocol whereby the nurses would prepare the patients, get all the supplies and medications for the epidural analgesia, and have the patient completely ready before the anesthesiologist arrived to place the epidural. According to this formalized work-around—including laminated reminder cards on the wall—nurses obtained the medication from the storage area without a physician's order to save time for the physician. When the physician came to the obstetrics unit, he or she then signed the orders for the drugs the nurse had pulled.

During her shift, the nurse was taking care of two patients: one whose child had died in utero but the patient had not yet given birth, and a 16-year-old having her first baby. Both of these patients required a lot of attention and compassion. The nurse was not only fatigued because of lack of sleep and long, back-to-back shifts, but she was dealing with emotionally charged patients, which was stressful. The teen needed an antibiotic to help treat a strep infection during labor. When the nurse went to hang the IV antibiotic, she accidentally hung a bag of local anesthetic—bupivicaine—which was housed in packaging that was very similar in appearance to the antibiotic. One drug had an orange dot on the bag. The other had a yellow dot. Both drugs were sitting on a table in the patient's room. The bupivicaine had been pulled by another nurse who was preparing to contact the anesthesiologist to give her patient an epidural.

Bupivicaine, a very commonly used local anesthetic, is very cardiotoxic, meaning that a significant IV dose can and will cause cardiac arrest. When the patient seized and suffered acute cardiovascular collapse, the care team emergently focused on getting down the hall to the operating room and delivering the baby by C-section. A normal baby was delivered. Unfortunately, the mother died.

As tragic as the death of a 16-year-old mother is, it was compounded by the fact that the nurse was now facing criminal charges in the patient's death. Despite the myriad system issues that led to the nurse's mistake—systematically encouraged fatigue, look-alike packaging, ineffective technology that led to work-arounds, and an approved process in which nurses pulled medication without a physician's order—the hospital did not view the death as a result of system failures but placed blame squarely on the shoulders of one of its finest nurses

In looking at this case objectively, how does blaming the nurse address the problem and prevent it from happening again? The fact is, it does not. Not only does this approach irrevocably alter the nurse's life and career, but it does not address the fundamental system issues that contributed to the mistake. It also eliminates the opportunity to learn from errors—both this one and any future errors—because staff members at the hospital know exactly how errors will be treated and what will happen to them if they admit a mistake.

In addition to the general ineffectiveness of blaming the conscientious employee who makes a mistake, another critically important side effect to this approach is that it creates and reinforces a culture of fear. In this environment, people learn quite quickly to be quiet about problems, mistakes, near misses, and the like because they expect punishment if they speak up. This in turn limits an organization's ability to learn from and address system errors. An adverse event provides insight into the care delivery process, and the open, honest discussion of adverse events is a primary way to truly understand the strengths and weaknesses of care delivery and opportunities for improving flawed policies and practices that increase the risk of error and patient harm.

DEFINING A JUST CULTURE

As mentioned in Chapter 1, one of the most important jobs of organization leadership is to foster a *just culture* in which everyone knows how the organization will view and respond to errors. It can be said that no other element plays as critical a role in defining a culture. A just culture is a culture of

trust in which people are encouraged to provide essential safety-related information, but in which they are also clear about where the line must be drawn between acceptable and unacceptable behavior.[1] Contrary to popular belief, establishing a just culture is not about removing blame. Removing blame from the workplace does not eliminate individual or organizational responsibility. A just culture is characterized by clear systems thinking, organizational learning, well-developed decision-making mechanisms, and clear organizational structures.[2]

According to one prominent health care organization, "A fair and just culture means giving constructive feedback and critical analysis in skillful ways, doing assessments that are based on facts, and having respect for the complexity of the situation. It also means providing fair-minded treatment, having productive conversations, and creating effective structures that help people reveal their errors and help the organization learn from them."[2(p. 619)]

A health care organization has established a "just culture" when the majority of its members share the belief that justice will be dispensed when the line between acceptable and unacceptable behavior has been crossed. A just culture recognizes that it is unacceptable to punish all errors and unsafe acts, and it is equally unacceptable to provide blanket immunity from sanctions to all actions that could, or did, contribute to harm.

Organizations that are successful in developing and sustaining a just culture are those that have a clear policy statement and framework to guide their response to unsafe acts and adverse outcomes, along with leadership's resolve to create a climate of "psychological safety"[3] and support caregivers who voice concerns.

ESTABLISHING AN ACCOUNTABILITY SYSTEM

To create and foster a just culture, leadership must define, communicate about, and consistently reinforce a system of accountability, which differentiates when good people inadvertently make a mistake because of a series of system issues and when individuals deliberately cause harm or knowingly put a patient at risk without sufficient potential benefit.

Individual accountability must be characterized by clear role definition and relationship delineation.[2] An accountability model enables an organization to promote a just culture that strikes a balance between the benefits of learning at the organizational, interpersonal, and individual levels and the need to retain personal accountability and discipline.[4]

Organizations should pledge within their policies to look objectively at errors and place blame appropriately. Staff members should know that they will be held accountable for their own performance but will not be expected to carry the burden for system flaws. They should know what to expect from the organization when an error occurs and how they will be held accountable. Staff should be assured that the constant goal is systems improvement and decreasing harm to the next patient, and that the act of speaking up will, first and foremost, be used to improve the system of care delivery.

WHY IS AN ACCOUNTABILITY SYSTEM IMPORTANT?

The main reason such an accountability system is critical is that people make mistakes. No matter how skilled, conscientious, well-intentioned, and experienced individuals may be, there are inherent human limitations or factors that make errors possible. Couple that with the fact that care, treatment, and services are often provided amid constant distractions when providers are tired, in a hurry, and under pressure, and individuals can overestimate their abilities and underestimate their limitations. They can fail to recognize the impact of factors such as fatigue, stress, and environmental distractions, including noise or poor lighting.

As mentioned in Chapter 1, the culture of many health care organizations is anchored by the belief that if skilled, smart people just try hard and work diligently, they can avoid mistakes and prevent human error. This model of the expert individual is strongly reinforced in the clinical education process. However, this viewpoint is inherently flawed, as humans by their very nature are wired to make mistakes, and no amount of hard work and effort can prevent that.

Errors of commission, such as administering the wrong medication to a patient because it looks or sounds like another; errors of omission, such as unknowingly skipping a step while programming a medication pump; and even simple arithmetic errors, which could happen, for example, when calculating a medication dose, are all part of the human condition and occur with alarming regularity. The fact is that people will forget to do something (error of omission) approximately 1 out of every 100 times they are required to do it. They will do something wrong (an error of commission) approximately 1 out of every 300 times.[5] Consider how many times a nurse must check a drug label in a typical day. Or how many times a physician must write an order for a particular drug. Or how many times a respiratory therapist must administer a particular medication. Now consider that 1 out of every 100–300 times that nurse will forget to read the label or read it incorrectly; that physician will leave something off of the prescription or write that prescription incorrectly; and that respiratory therapist may forget to administer a medication or administer it incorrectly. How will your organization react to these errors? How you answer that question will help define whether you have a just culture or not.

Factors That Negatively Affect Human Performance

There are many human factors that lead to error in the health care environment. For example, illness, boredom, frustration, and the use of drugs and alcohol can all impair performance and lead to human error. The following sections take a brief look at some of the other human factors that can lead to error:

• Limited short-term memory. The human brain can hold only five to seven pieces of information in short-term memory at one time. Practitioners in a complex environment like medicine deal with a continuous yet frequently interrupted flow of information and tasks over the course of a day—often on a minute-to-minute basis. In fact, observational studies of medical/surgical nurses show that they are trying to hold 17–20 items in memory 70% of the time they are at work.[6] Being in a busy environment with information constantly coming in means that an individual's ability to hold, keep track of, prioritize, and manage all the information being received is quickly exceeded. Systems that rely on human memory are highly prone to failure.

• Being late or in a hurry. It is human nature to cut corners when behind or in a hurry. The great majority of the time, cutting corners pays off. The job gets done more quickly or is a little bit easier, and there is no apparent downside because errors are rare and the impact of many errors is modest. In fact, individuals are typically rewarded for cutting corners. However, when in a hurry, a person is less selective in his or her attention to details, and the chances of missing something that can contribute to error and possibly cause harm increase significantly. There is a very real danger with cutting corners that over time progressively more corners will be cut without any apparent compromise of safety. The cumulative effect of all these cut corners is called the "normalization of deviance"—when things that are obviously risky become accepted as "we've always done it that way and never had a problem."[7] (See Sidebar 3-1, right, for a further discussion of normalization of deviance.)

• Limited ability to multitask. Most people, even highly trained ones, are not good multitaskers. Typically, individuals are far better at singular task performance. An example of this is people's inability to drive cars safely and talk on cell phones. According to the National Safety Council assessment in 2011, at least 23% of all traffic crashes—or at least 1.3 million crashes per year—involve cell phone use.[8]

In health care, providers—particularly nurses—are asked to multitask every day. They must check for allergies and administer medication to one patient, while changing a dressing on another patient, while taking vital signs on another patient, and also remember to regularly wash their hands, document information, and communicate effectively. According to a study by Tucker and Spear, nurses perform an average of 100 tasks in an eight-hour shift, with each task taking an average of three minutes. They spend time running from task to task to task, and often don't know what the overall plan of care is and thus have a limited ability to prioritize. They are also formally interrupted at least once every hour. As a result of this environment, when a patient has a problem, the nurse is so busy multitasking, he or she may not notice the issue until it has reached a critical level.[9]

• Interruptions. The daily experience in complex environments like medicine is that interruptions are more the norm than the exception. When distracted from tasks considered critically important, even experts require formal cues to get back on track. Interruptions are a huge source of risk, and yet they tend to be regarded as annoyances rather than as the threat they pose. When interrupted, an individual's ability to get back on task is dependent on short-term memory, which, as previously discussed, is quite limited.

• Stress. Human factors research consistently demonstrates that error rates increase with significant stress. Individuals have a 30% chance of making an error when highly stressed, as opposed to a 0.1% chance when not

Sidebar 3-1.
The Normalization of Deviance

The normalization of deviance is a term authored by Diane Vaughan in her analysis of the 1986 *Challenger* space shuttle accident. It refers to the accumulated effect of cutting corners over time. While the effect of each of these shortcuts individually is usually not significant, when added together, what is considered safe and reasonable can be changed dramatically. Very typically, the normalization of deviance leaves everyone shaking their heads in the aftermath of an accident and asking, "How did we get here?"

In the case of the *Challenger* disaster, over a period of 24 launches in the NASA Shuttle program, the minimum safe launch temperature incrementally moved from 55 degrees Fahrenheit to 36 degrees on the January day in 1986 when the O-rings failed. Slowly, over time, these numerous small reductions in the safe launch temperature pushed the envelope of safety.

The loss of the *Columbia* space shuttle in 2003 resulted from a similar problem. During many previous shuttle flights, foam insulation fell from the external fuel tank during liftoff. These flights were seemingly unaffected by the debris and thus the problem was ignored. Unfortunately, on February 1, 2003, the falling insulation damaged the shuttle's left wing and was the physical cause of the tragedy. According to the *Chicago Tribune*, the pressure to keep on schedule led NASA to habitually accept the persistent problem of the falling foam and come to view it as normal.

Though the technical term Vaughan applied to the *Challenger* launch decision was "The Normalization of Deviance," a common, practical term to describe the accumulated result of many shortcuts is "drift."

Sources: Vaughan D. *The Challenger Launch Decision: Risky Technology, Culture, and Deviance at NASA.* Chicago: University of Chicago Press, 1996; Leonard M, Frankel A. Focusing on high reliability. In Leonard M, Frankel A, Simmonds T, editors: *Achieving Safe and Reliable Healthcare: Strategies and Solutions.* Chicago: Health Administration Press, 2004, 15–34; Kunerth J, Cabbage M. NASA's safety culture blamed. *Chicago Tribune.* 2003 Aug 27:1, 26.

stressed. When under stress, there is an increased likelihood that individuals will shift from rapid, accurate expert decision making to an inefficient, slow, conscious problem-solving process that is highly error-prone. For example, under normal circumstances, a provider can successfully select and pick out the correct medication vial 99.9% of the time. However, when performing the same task in a very stressful situation, such as the middle of a cardiac arrest, the error rate can be as high as 25%, a 250-fold increase![5]

Stress is also a likely contributor toward tunnel vision—not being able to see the forest for the trees. People who are stressed can easily become "tunnel-visioned" and lose sight of the bigger picture. They also tend to revert to previous patterns of behavior and are more likely to filter information in ways that fit the desired end result. This tendency greatly increases the chances that conclusions are wrong. If an individual makes the wrong choice initially, the danger is that he or she will selectively filter incoming information to verify his or her initial decision, and discard critical data that reveal something else is going on.

Consider this unfortunate (and true) example: An anesthesiologist is putting a healthy patient to sleep. Everything is going smoothly, and the anesthesiologist is easily ventilating the patient using a mask. However, when the endotracheal breathing tube is placed, the patient has extreme difficulty breathing. The pressure required to deliver a breath is alarmingly high; the end-tidal CO_2 monitor—the gold standard used to verify the integrity of a patient's breathing—reads zero; and the patient's oxygen saturation falls to life-threatening levels. Not considering the possibility that the breathing tube is in the wrong place—the leading cause of anesthetic death in healthy patients—the physician interprets the situation as an indicator of an acute, massive asthma attack. The absence of carbon dioxide on the monitor is attributed to abrupt failure of the device, which has worked well for the anesthesiologist on three prior cases that day.

In reality, the patient's breathing tube has been mistakenly placed in the esophagus, and the anesthesiologist, not recognizing the potentially lethal error, persists in reading the incoming data into his very tenuous construct. The critical error in this case is not placing the tube incorrectly—it happens to the best of clinicians—but not recognizing the problem and fixing it. If the anesthesiologist had thought, "Things were great until the tube was placed, and then the problem began. Let's take the tube out and see if things get better," this situation would have been a nonevent. However, the failure to consider a possible mistake and the refusal to interpret overwhelmingly obvious information indicating that the tube is in the wrong place does great harm.[7]

• Lack of sleep and fatigue. Sleepiness can be defined as a tendency to fall asleep, whereas fatigue is an overwhelming sense of tiredness, lack of energy, and a feeling of exhaustion accompanied by impaired physical and/or cognitive functioning.[10] Fatigue can result from lack of sleep, illness, vigorous exercise, or prolonged concentration. Each

year, millions of Americans progress through life fatigued. Nearly 40% of the workforce experiences fatigue on the job,[11] and nearly 70% of the public does not get enough sleep during the week.[12] In the often fast-paced world of health care, worker fatigue has always been a potential patient safety and provider safety risk. It has been linked to decreases in performance and increases in medical errors and workplace accidents.

Fatigue can have a detrimental effect on cognitive ability, specifically the ability to process complex information. The working assumption that motivation and skill can overcome inherent physiologic limitations of fatigue is a dangerous one. It has been shown that cognitive performance after 24 hours without sleep is equivalent to performance with a blood alcohol level of 0.10.[13] Research also shows that sleep debt is cumulative and the physiologic effects will persist until enough sleep has been obtained to pay it back.[14] A chronically sleep-restricted individual may have a false sense of recovery; an ability to perform well for the first several hours can mask the effects of chronic sleep loss during a typical waking day.[15]

Fatigue can affect physicians' and nurses' technical skills and their ability to perform specific procedures. For example, studies have shown that surgeons have less surgical dexterity and operate more slowly when fatigued.[16] Whether administering an IV medication or monitoring a patient during anesthesia, degradation of attention, memory, and coordination due to fatigue can affect performance, affect patient safety, and lead to adverse events.[17] Mistakes caused by fatigue are most likely to occur during routine tasks and those that require sustained concentration. Effects on urgent tasks or those that require short yet significant bursts of mental energy are less. Often, fatigue-related mistakes involve the failure to recognize the existence of a serious problem. For example, giving the wrong antibiotic to a septic patient is not typically a fatigue-related mistake; however, failing to recognize that altered mental status might represent sepsis is typical of a fatigue-related error.[18]

Interestingly enough, fatigue causes fewer performance problems in workers with more control over their work because they can schedule nonurgent tasks or tasks that require sustained concentration for periods when they are at their best. Physicians will thus cope better with fatigue than staff members with less job flexibility, such as nurses.[18]

In addition to the patient safety risks associated with

fatigue, there are several provider safety risks. Physical and mental health, interpersonal relationships, and the ability to perform the tasks of daily life can all be affected by acute sleep loss and fatigue. In addition to detrimental health effects, there is a well-documented connection between fatigue and an increased likelihood of on-the-job accidents.[19] Some of those accidents may include needlestick injuries and bloodborne pathogen exposure. One study found that the number of hours worked per day, the number of weekends worked per month, and whether individuals worked evening and night shifts were significantly associated with needlestick injuries.[20]

Fatigue is not only a contributor to workplace accidents but accidents that occur outside the workplace as well. According to one study, first-year medical interns who work shifts longer than 24 hours are more than twice as likely as interns who work shorter shifts to be in a car crash after leaving work, and five times as likely to have a near-miss (close call).[21] Studies also report increased rates of crashes in nurses when driving home after working a night shift.[22] Another study showed that 24% of residents surveyed reported falling asleep driving home since becoming a physician, 66% had felt close to falling asleep at the wheel in the past 12 months, and 42% recalled a fatigue-related clinical error in the previous 6 months.[23]

• The detrimental effects of shift work. Hospitals function around the clock and therefore require shift work. Typically, shift work is performed outside the daytime hours of 7 A.M. to 6 P.M. and includes evening shifts, night shifts, rotating shifts, and on-call shifts. More than 20% of the workforce in the United States participates in shift work, and approximately 30% of nurses employed in full-time health care engage in this type of work.[24] In health care, individuals who participate in shift work or who engage in prolonged work hours—such as shifts lasting 12 hours or more—are more likely to be fatigued than those who work a more regular schedule. Evening and night-shift workers can be particularly susceptible to fatigue. Human beings are biologically wired to be awake during the day and asleep at night, and work schedules that oppose this natural rhythm can generate physiologic disruptions that lead to significantly degraded performance and increased risks to health and safety.[25] Physicians-in-training who work traditional schedules with recurrent 24-hour shifts greatly increase the risk of injuring their patients or others and incur the follow-

ing risks[26]:

• Make 36% more serious medical errors than those whose scheduled work is limited to 15 consecutive hours

• Make five times as many serious diagnostic errors

• Have twice as many on-the-job attention failures at night

• Suffer 61% more needlestick and other sharps injuries after 20 consecutive hours of work

• Report making 300% more fatigue-related medical errors that lead to a patient's death

In one study, in which residents were surveyed about medical errors, the odds of reporting at least one fatigue-related clinically significant medical error increased by a factor of 7 during months in which the residents worked five or more overnight shifts, as compared with months in which they worked no overnight shifts.[27] The study showed that interns made 35.9% more serious medical errors when they worked frequent shifts of 24 hours or more—a more traditional schedule—than when they worked shorter shifts. They also made 56.6% more nonintercepted serious errors and 5.6 times as many serious diagnostic errors during the traditional schedule. Consequently, the study showed that eliminating extended work shifts and reducing the number of hours interns work per week can reduce serious medical errors.[27]

Nurses encounter similar shift work–related fatigue risks. A study of nurses showed that the risk of a nurse making an error significantly increased when the nurse's work shift exceeded 12 hours, when overtime was worked, or when work hours exceeded more than 40 hours per week. In fact, the likelihood of a nurse making an error was three times higher when the shift lasted 12.5 hours or more. This study also indicated that many nurses work past their scheduled shift time, and those individuals who did work past their 12-hour shift were most vulnerable for making an error.[28]

• Environmental factors. Environmental factors, such as heat, noise, visual stimuli, distractions, and lighting, can all adversely affect human performance and lead to mistakes. Environmental distractions can be seen in operating rooms, which are frequently noisy with music playing, patient monitors beeping, and conversations going on. In addition, there are electrical cords on the floor, and various tubes and gas lines are present. From an ergonomic engineering point of view, the array, or more appropriately, disarray of equipment, is a chaotic nightmare. In addition, many operating room doors are barely wide enough to accommodate a patient bed going in or out. Workplace design is an integral part of keeping patients and staff safe.

System Errors and Latent Failures

In addition to human factors that lead to human error, system malfunctions, limitations, and breakdowns can also lead to error. Also know as "latent errors," these might include poorly designed work flow, incorrect installation of equipment, faulty maintenance, and poor organizational structure. In health care, frontline providers are so used to design defects resulting from latent errors that they learn to work around them. These work-arounds can also lead to error because safety steps are often skipped or overlooked. It is essential to have a good understanding of complex systems and of latent and active failures when building a model of accountability. James Reason's work is an excellent place to start.[1] Both human and latent system errors do not always lead to harm. Many times providers will notice problems in situations and address them before they cause harm. Other errors do reach the patient, but, because of the resiliency of the human body among other factors, don't cause harm. However, the combination of human factors and system issues can sometimes create the "perfect storm" in health care, with the patient in the eye of the storm. It is in this perfect storm that we see a majority of preventable adverse outcomes, and it is the navigation of this storm that requires an accountability system.

HOW TO CREATE A JUST ACCOUNTABILITY SYSTEM

Creating an accountability system does not have to be challenging. Although there are many ways to create such a system, one easy way is to base it on James Reason's five-part algorithm,[1] which involves asking the following questions whenever an error occurs:

1. Was there malicious intent? Did the individual intentionally engage in activity to cause harm?

2. Was the person knowingly impaired? For example, was he or she intoxicated or under the influence of an unauthorized substance, such as illicit drugs? Was there a medical illness that impaired his or her judgment?

3. Did the individual do something he or she knew was wrong or knowingly unsafe? For example, was the person

knowingly violating safe operating procedure, such as refusing to engage in a presurgical time-out to verify the correct patient, procedure, and site?

4. Did the individual make a mistake someone of similar training would make? For example, if a patient in the emergency department has a grossly abnormal electrocardiogram, and the physician sends him home where he suffers a heart attack and dies, the question becomes would another physician have made the same mistake given the system issues present at the time?

5. Is the individual involved a "frequent flier"—has he or she been involved in multiple adverse events? Has he or she been repeatedly involved in similar events?

Within Reason's model, the first three components reveal violations at an individual level and indicate that the individual should be held accountable for his or her actions. The fourth question is sometimes referred to as the substitution test and can indicate whether there is an individual issue or a system error. If two to three peers would make a similar mistake given the circumstances, then the error can be attributed to system issues. However, if an individual's peers would not make such a mistake then it raises questions of technical skill, training, and judgment.

The fifth question, which deals with repeat participants, raises significant issues as to judgment and knowledge.

Can these be mitigated with training and education? People who have been involved multiple times in similar events are less likely to be good candidates for training and education. If an organization concludes that these types of interventions do not have a likelihood of success, they do have a nonnegotiable obligation to provide safe care. In these instances, these individuals may need to be changed to a different role.

Let's go back to the example at the beginning of this chapter. In asking the five questions about the veteran nurse who made a mistake, which led to the death of a teenage girl, how would you classify the error?

- Was there malicious intent? Did the nurse intentionally engage in activity to cause harm? No.

- Was the nurse knowingly impaired? For example, was she intoxicated or under the influence of an unauthorized substance, such as illicit drugs? Was there a medical illness that impaired her judgment? No.

- Did the individual do something she knew was wrong or knowingly unsafe? Although the nurse did obtain drugs without a physician's order, this was tacitly sanctioned by the organization as part of a performance improvement initiative. Did she engage in conscious risk taking by not using the bar-coding system? We would need to know whether it was available and working, and how many other nurses were working around it. If this was common behavior on the unit, it is hard to hold one nurse accountable. If she was the only one, that changes the conversation.

• Did the individual make a mistake someone of similar training would make? Yes. If one of her peers was fatigued, stressed, in a hurry, working around a poorly functioning technology, and following a protocol that was inherently flawed just as this nurse was, the likelihood the peer would make the same mistake is great.

• Had she been involved in similar events? No.

Although James Reason's model is not the only way to establish an accountability system, it provides a clear-cut and straightforward way to start the process. By incorporating some version of Reason's algorithm into your organization's accountability system, you can deal with most accountability questions very quickly. It is critically important that the caregiver at the bedside be able to ask himself or herself a very short list of questions in the aftermath of an error or near miss to determine his or her level of accountability and know it is safe to tell someone about the event, so the situation can likely be remedied to prevent it from happening again. It is also important that the organization has only "one set of rules," applied consistently and openly to everyone regardless of their standing in the organization or the severity of the event.

In addition to Reason's model, David Marx, an engineer and lawyer, elegantly applied an engineering perspective to accountability and developed a Just Culture Algorithm, which has become popular in the United States. The algorithm has as its foundation the concept that individuals should be held accountable for the choices they make. Marx has taken this tack because the provision of health care, particularly among physicians, has tended toward a perspective of "no harm, no foul"—in other words even if an action is reckless, if no damage occurs, organizations are willing to turn a blind eye to the activity.[4]

Marx divides actions into three categories to support this framework. Actions deemed blameless occur when individuals inadvertently make mistakes or errors. The causes of these errors have been aptly described in this chapter and are a result of human fallibility, especially in complex environments.

The algorithm then delves into an aspect of decision making that Reason's indecision tree hints at in his substitution test—when he asks whether other similarly skilled and trained individuals would perform in the same way as the individual being evaluated—but the substitution test only touches on at a concept that Marx goes into in great detail. Marx describes the other two categories of actions as "at-risk" behavior and "reckless" behavior and is quick to point out that differentiation between the two can be made only through the lens of what the culture—the local society—perceives as allowable. An example helps to clarify this nuanced issue. Take hand washing. Today, most would agree that choosing to not wash hands prior to touching a patient is blatant reckless behavior. Indeed, if the hospital deems hand hygiene noncompliance as reckless and responds accordingly by uniform sanctions when noncompliance occurs, individuals will be on notice to carefully wash their hands, and other than the occasional mistake where a clinician forgets or is distracted while entering a patient's room (both blameless and allowable omission errors), exceptions to good hand washing will be forbidden and noncompliance will be, to all, reckless behavior. However, if a hospital deems hand hygiene noncompliance as reckless yet doesn't respond when individuals knowingly ignore the rules, then, by cultural norm, omitting washing hands is "at-risk" behavior. Organizations that then arbitrarily sanction clinicians only by outcome, when patients become infected, are acting erratically—and destined to be perceived by their employees and clinicians as untrustworthy. The effect is to stymie efforts that promote transparency and learning because individuals are unsure of the response they'll receive. The clinician is accountable for at-risk behavior, and the organization is accountable for poorly upholding its standards of care.

Marx describes a just culture as one that "recognizes that while we as humans are fallible, we do generally have control of our behavioral choices, whether we are an executive, a manager, or a staff member. Just culture flourishes in an organization that understands the concept of shared accountability—that good system design and good behavioral choices of staff together produce good results. It has to be both."[29(p. 1)]

RELENTLESSLY REINFORCE THE MESSAGE

Before implementing an accountability system, it may be helpful to determine the staff's familiarity with the concept of a nonpunitive culture. Both frontline staff and managers must be clear on what is expected from them and how they will be held accountable for errors.

After leaders have established an accountability system, they can't just mention it once and forget it, they must continuously educate, reinforce, and demonstrate their commitment to consistent accountability and learning from mistakes. This can't be stressed enough. Because accountability is a critical element in the creation and maintenance of a safe culture, organization leadership must commit to an accountability system and consistent application of that system across the organization. Some ways to do this include the following:

• Create policies and procedures that support the accountability system and the entire error management process. Such policies should be shared with staff and leadership.

• Educate frontline staff on the accountability system. This education needs to be wall-to-wall. All staff should be educated on the policy and see consistent reinforcement of it by leadership. Education can take many forms, including during staff meetings, within WalkRounds (*see* Chapter 5), during online training sessions, and so forth. Such education should change these staff perspectives:

—That was a weak moment. I won't do it again.

—I am absolutely not going to tell anyone, because I will get in big trouble.

—Why should I tell them? Nothing will change.

• Educate staff on human factors and their contributions to medical error. This type of education must combat the previously mentioned cultural tendency to assume that through hard work and commitment, errors can be avoided. Staff members should be aware of the human factors that contribute to error and be able to recognize those factors in their work life. They also should feel comfortable reporting situations in which human factors have the potential to cause errors and work to redesign processes to mitigate the effects of those factors. For example, to help combat the effects of fatigue, some organizations are instituting a planned nap program for individuals who work the night shift. In most cases, the nap is voluntary. Staff must learn the effects of fatigue on performance, recognize the signs of fatigue, and feel empowered to take a planned nap when necessary.

• Make the accountability system part of the orientation process for new hires as well as the continuing education program for current staff.

• Educate managers on the accountability system. Middle management must understand the algorithm, know how to use it, and be held accountable for using it consistently. Your organization may want to use scenarios or case examples to help train managers so that they can get practice in consistently using the algorithm. If an event does not neatly fit within the algorithm, managers should be supported with a senior-level management group that helps navigate gray areas.

• Use real case examples to both educate and reinforce the accountability model—the best ones are your own events. Real cases are very powerful, as many clinicians will have already heard about the event through the rumor mill, and this is a golden opportunity for leaders to model the desired approach to analyzing these events. Not only does it show consistency, it also teaches people about system error and illustrates the organizational commitment to safe care.

• Senior leadership must publicly embrace the accountability system and hold middle management accountable for using it. In a case in which a high-profile error goes public, senior leadership must support the participants in the error and avoid the temptation to place blame.

• Create a process in which you learn from errors. As previously mentioned, adverse events provide a unique opportunity for learning. After an event occurs and it is determined to be a system error, your organization should have a consistent process of learning from that error. This should involve looking at contributing factors, such as human factors, environmental considerations, faulty equipment, and so forth. Often, organizations will use a root cause analysis for this process, which is a step-by-step approach to analyzing an error, determining the primary cause(s) of the error, and working to put improvements in place to address the error. More information about root cause analysis can be found in Chapter 12.

As previously mentioned, a key element in an effective accountability system is consistency. The system must be applied the same way every time there is an error. It takes only one case in which a CEO places blame on a frontline provider for a system error, and the entire accountability system and culture of safety is seriously jeopardized as a result of the fragile trust built between staff and leadership being shattered.

A good accountability model is the essential foundation of a functional and safe organizational culture. When caregivers know that there is a transparent set of rules that apply to everyone, and that roughly 95% of the time following an adverse event the individuals involved are recognized as conscientious, highly skilled individuals trying hard to do the right thing, then caregivers will know they are safe to report and discuss errors. This transparency and accountability also allow your organization to say to staff, patients and families, the media, and regulators that the people who provide care in your organization are capable, conscientious, and trying very hard to do the right things for every patient every day. It is absolutely essential for caregivers to feel safe; otherwise, they never really believe the organization can keep patients safe.

REFERENCES

1. Reason J. *Managing the Risks of Organizational Accidents.* Burlington, VT: Ashgate, 1997.
2. Connor M, et al. Creating a fair and just culture: One organization's path toward organizational change. *Jt Comm J Qual Patient Saf.* 2007;33(10):617–624.
3. Edmondson AC. The competitive imperative of learning. *Harv Bus Rev.* 2008;86(7–8):60–67.
4. Marx D. *Patient Safety and the "Just Culture": A Primer for Health Care Executives.* New York City: Columbia University, 2001.
5. Salvendy G. *Handbook of Human Factors and Ergonomics,* 3rd ed. Hoboken, NJ: Wiley, 2006.
6. Potter P, et al. Understanding the cognitive work of nursing in the acute care environment. *J Nurs Adm.* 2005;35(7–8):327–335.
7. Leonard M, Frankel A. Focusing on high reliability. In Leonard M, Frankel A, Simmonds T, editors: *Achieving Safe and Reliable Healthcare: Strategies and Solutions.* Chicago: Health Administration Press, 2004, 15–34.
8. National Safety Council. Press Release: National Safety Council Estimates That at Least 1.6 Million Crashes Each Year Involve Drivers Using Cell Phones and Texting. Jan 12, 2010. (Updated: 2011.) Accessed Oct 30, 2012. http://www.nsc.org/Pages/NSCestimates 16millioncrashescausedbydriversusingcellphonesandtexting.aspx.
9. Tucker AL, Spear SJ. Operational failures and interruptions in hospital nursing. *Health Serv Res.* 2006;41(3 Pt 1):643–662.
10. Shen J, Barbera J, Shapiro CM. Distinguishing sleepiness and fatigue: Focus on definition and measurement. *Sleep Med Rev.* 2006;10(1):63–76.
11. Medical News Today. Fatigue in the Workplace Is Common and Costly. Jan 15, 2007. Accessed Octo 30, 2012. http://www.medicalnewstoday.com/medicalnews.php?newsid=60732.
12. National Sleep Foundation. *2002 "Sleep in America" Poll.* Washington, DC: National Sleep Foundation, Mar 2002. Accessed Oct 30, 2012. http://www.sleepfoundation.org/sites/default/files/2002SleepInAmericaPoll.pdf.
13. Baker A, Simpson S, Dawson D. Sleep disruption and mood changes associated with menopause. *J Psychosom Res.* 1997;43(4):359–369.
14. Dinges DF. Sleep debt and scientific evidence. *Sleep.* 2004 Sep 15;27(6):1050–1052.
15. Cohen DA, et al. Uncovering residual effects of chronic sleep loss on human performance. *Sci Transl Med.* 2010 Jan 13;2(14):14ra3.
16. Eastridge BJ, et al. Effect of sleep deprivation on the performance of simulated laparoscopic surgical skill. *Am J Surg.* 2003;186(2):169–174.
17. Jha AK, Duncan BW, Bates DW. Fatigue, sleepiness, and medical errors. In Shojania KG, et al., editors: *Making Health Care Safer: A Critical Analysis of Patient Safety Practices.* Evidence Report/Technology Assessment No. 43. Rockville, MD: Agency for Healthcare Research and Quality, 2001, 519–532. Accessed Oct 20, 2012. http://www.ahrq.gov/clinic/ptsafety/chap46a.htm.
18. Olson LG, Ambrogetti A. Working harder—Working dangerously? Fatigue and performance in hospitals. *Med J Aust.* 1998 Jun 15;168(12):614–616.
19. ECRI Patient Safety Center. Fatigue in healthcare workers. HRC Supplement A: Risk Analysis Employment Issues 14. ECRI. Jan 2006.
20. Trinkoff AM, et al. Work schedule, needle use, and needlestick injuries among registered nurses. *Infect Control Hosp Epidemiol.* 2007;28(2):156–164.
21. Barger LK, et al.; Harvard Work Hours, Health, and Safety Group. Extended work shifts and the risk of motor vehicle crashes among interns. *N Engl J Med.* 2005 Jan 13;352(2):125–134.
22. Caruso CC, Condon ME. Night shifts and fatigue: Coping skills for the working nurse. *Am J Nurs.* 2006;106(8):88.
23. Gander P, et al. Work patterns and fatigue-related risk among junior doctors. *Occup Environ Med.* 2007;64(11):733–738.
24. Blachowicz E, Letizia M. The challenges of shift work. *Medsurg Nurs.* 2006;15(5):274–280.
25. Rosekind MR. Managing work schedules: An alertness and safety perspective. In Kryger MA, Roth T, Dement WC, editors: *Principles and Practice of Sleep Medicine,* 4th ed. Philadelphia: Elsevier Saunders, 2005, 680–690.
26. Lockley SW, et al. Effects of health care provider work hours and sleep deprivation on safety and performance. *Jt Comm J Qual Patient Saf.* 2007;33(11 Suppl):7–18.
27. Barger LK, et al. Impact of extended-duration shifts on medical errors, adverse events, and attentional failures. *PLoS Med.* 2006;3(12):e487.
28. Rogers AE, et al. The working hours of hospital staff nurses and patient safety. *Health Aff (Millwood).* 2004;23(4):202–212.
29. Marx D, Comden SC, Sexhus Z. Our inaugural issue—In recognition of a growing community. *The Just Culture Community News and Views.* 2005;(1):1.

Chapter Four

RELIABILITY AND RESILIENCE

Roger Resar, MD; Frank Federico, RPh; Doug Bonacum, MBA, BS; Carol Haraden, PhD

ealth care is one of the most complex systems in existence. Within the health care system, multiple specialized disciplines interact with each other as well as with sophisticated equipment to perform complex procedures in a fast-paced environment. Both the number and type of interacting factors at play can be mind boggling, and the way health care is provided can change from day to day and patient to patient. The complexity and lack of predictability inherent in health care places a premium on reliability—both in processes and in the overall goals of an organization.

WHAT IS RELIABILITY?

In simplest terms, *reliability* is the probability that a system will consistently perform as designed over time. It's putting your key in the ignition of your car and being certain it will start; it's knowing that the newspaper is going to be delivered to your door without your having to do anything; it's turning on the TV at night and knowing the news will start exactly at the top of the hour.

Berwick and Nolan defined reliability for health care as "the capability of a process, procedure, or health service to perform its intended function in the required time under commonly existing conditions."[1] In terms of the aspirations of most health care organizations today, reliability is about providing the right care, to the right patient, at the right time . . . every time. Although this may seem obvious, McGlynn et al. have reported that patients actually receive only about an average of 55% of the "right" care and preventive therapy that they should.[2] For example, a process with 16 steps, each step interdependent on the other, would yield an overall level of reliability of 49% even if each step were 95.7% reliable! This is calculated by multiplying 95.7% by itself 16 times, yielding 49%. Considering the complexity of most health care work flows, it is no wonder that it is so difficult to

deliver all the "right" care and preventive therapy to patients. The importance of this concept in these calculations provides greater understanding into how to achieve high levels of reliability in the face of intrinsic human limitations and error rates—simplify processes by reducing the number of steps.

The reliability of a process or system can be thought of as the opposite of its rate of error or failure. For example, when a system has an error rate of 1 in 10, it is operating at a level of reliability of 90%. When the error or defect rate is 1 in 100, the level of reliability is 99%. For many processes in health care, achieving an overall reliability rate of approximately 95% would result in remarkably more patient-centered, effective, and efficient care. For other processes, however, such as administering medication, even a 99% rate of reliability would be disastrous. In the labeling of laboratory specimens, a 99.9% success rate is inadequate to safeguard patients.

WHY DO ORGANIZATIONS STRUGGLE WITH RELIABILITY?

With all the good intentions and talent available in health care, why are clinical processes that are backed by solid medical evidence carried out at such low levels of reliability? Certainly, few people come to work with the intention of performing poorly. The following common themes may offer a partial explanation for the reliability gap:

- Low-impact changes that emphasize vigilance and hard work. Current improvement methods in health care depend excessively on asking people to "pay more attention," "slow down," and "try harder." As discussed in Chapter 3, humans make mistakes, and asking them to pay more attention or try harder won't prevent that from happening. This approach is akin to asking yourself not to forget where you put your car keys or where you parked in a large parking lot. While it may be effective every once in awhile, you are still likely to misplace your keys or forget where you parked your car on some occasions, no matter how hard you try.

• Focus on individual clinician outcomes. The focus on individual clinician outcomes tends to exaggerate reliability. As discussed in Chapter 1, one reason that high error rates exist may be a lack of individual practitioner awareness of the problem. Although error rates are substantial, injuries due to error are not part of the everyday experience of physicians and nurses, and most errors do no harm—they are either intercepted through another individual's vigilance, often the patients, or if they do reach the patient by serendipity, their effects are nil or minor. For example, few children die from a single misdiagnosed or mistreated urinary infection, and many times nurses don't completely follow the "five rights" of medication administration, yet their patients still get the right dose of the right medication via the right route at the right time. When improvement programs are launched and aimed at decreasing the error rate by improving the reliability of the care process in question, clinicians often are skeptical. The quoted error rate does not match their reality. It is only when the reliability of the process is measured and shared that clinicians may begin to understand the problem.

• The toxicity of benchmarking. Organizations often benchmark against others in their peer group and feel secure when they fall within the same performance range. However, the entire peer group may have suboptimal performance, and comparison to that group does not help the organization understand the gap between their performance and the best possible outcome. When organizations compare themselves to top-performing organizations, they can more clearly see how their performance needs to improve.

• Lack of focus on process reliability. When there is a focus on bad outcomes and they are rare, there is the false sense of security that systems must be reliable, otherwise there would be more bad outcomes.

• Excessive clinical autonomy. Clinical autonomy allows wide performance margins. Autonomy, described by Reinertsen,[3] is that which stands between the great respect for evidence-based medicine and its implementation. In many health care organizations, clinicians have different approaches to care and prefer to be autonomous in how they provide care. One significant consequence of autonomy is unnecessary variation. Unnecessary variation adds complexity to an already complex system, complexity adds ambiguity, and ambiguity creates gaps between what we know and what we do. Unfortunately, our passion for fixing the problem is often trumped by a passion to fight for autonomy, so improvement is severely limited. Note that autonomy is not just an issue for physicians, it also applies to clinicians at all levels of care.

• Normalization of deviance. As discussed in Chapter 3, Vaughan, in describing the space shuttle *Challenger* disaster, coined the term *normalization of deviance*, as a long-term phenomenon in which individuals or teams repeatedly "get away" with a departure from established standards.[4] Thought process is dominated by this logic: Repeated success in accepting deviance from established standards implies future success. Over time, the individual/team fails to see their actions as deviant. In health care, normalization of deviance is often called "drift" from safe practice. Process reliability is always at risk from "drift." Drift leads to "predictable surprises," which are invariably disastrous to the patient, and secondarily, to the involved practitioners. These "predictable surprises" are often mislabeled "unanticipated adverse outcomes," but the fact that they are predictable means that they can be minimized through good engineering design and teamwork.

• Ineffective approaches to error reduction. In the aftermath of "predictable surprises," organizations fail to respond to errors in a manner that prevents recurrence. Errors come to be viewed as serious professional failures, the perception being that the individual "wasn't careful enough." There is little understanding of the design of reliable processes that can reduce the opportunity for errors. The misguided concept of infallibility inhibits learning from mistakes, creates fear, and results in corrective action that includes a lot of hand-wringing from management regarding what the practitioner "should have" done. Rarely are the systemic factors that drove the adverse outcome identified and mitigated in a way that dramatically reduces the probability or severity of incident recurrence.

• Lack of specific and measureable reliability targets. Processes are rarely designed to meet specific goals. Often organizations redesign processes with no specific goals for performance of the process. When designing a process it's important to set clear targets for reliability. For example, stating that a new process is going to work 95% of the time is an appropriate reliability target because achieving 95%

reliability is a reachable goal that doesn't necessarily require significant resources or technology.

DESIGNING FOR RELIABILITY

A first step in achieving reliability in your organization is to design and implement reliable processes and systems. Industries in which many lives rest upon performing every single task that is required, again and again, such as airlines and nuclear power plants, are famous for designing high-reliability processes and systems. Reliable design assists in preventing behaviors and conditions that lead to harm by creating an articulated and workable process that is readily followed and prevents conditions that increase risk due to human factors issues.

To help with reliable design, the Institute for Healthcare Improvement (IHI) has created an approach to redesigning daily work flows that can serve as a foundation to prevent harm from occurring as a result of error. The following sections discuss IHI's approach.

The Prep Work

Prior to redesigning for reliability, there are some "setup" steps required. Failure to set up improvement or redesign projects properly will, at best, delay meaningful change by months, but may, at worst, doom the project. The first step is to select a process that is noncatastrophic to improve. This means that failure to reliably carry out this process does not lead to patient death or serious injury within a short time period. A noncatastrophic process could be the delivery of preoperative antibiotics. Although potentially harmful if not done reliably, imminent death or serious harm to the patient is not a foregone conclusion. Conversely, operating on the wrong surgical site would be a catastrophic error because after the error occurs there is no way it can be undone, and irrevocable harm or death is ensured. Any clinical practice that is so critical that failure would lead to certain death or serious disability must be redesigned in a more robust way, such as by using Six Sigma methodology. (*See* Chapter 12 for more information on Six Sigma.) Other examples of processes that can result in catastrophic outcomes include the administration of blood and chemotherapy.

After a process has been selected, the improvement team must choose a segment of the process on which to test redesigns. It is important when segmenting to choose a segment that has a high enough volume so that study of changes reaps adequate information for analysis. Rapid testing offers the best opportunities for learning. The volume of the segment must be large enough that an improvement team can test daily or every other day. The speed of learning will be limited if the volume is so low that teams cannot test frequently. For example, if the improvement team is testing a new checklist and can test only once a week, it will take many weeks before the team can learn and improve the process. On the other hand, if there is an opportunity to test daily or every other day, the improvement team will have opportunities to learn and improve more quickly. The chosen segment should also provide a high probability of success for the types of changes that may be tested. For example, it may be appropriate and helpful to test a process on a particular unit or units, a particular patient population, or a particular aspect of the process.

After selecting a segment, your organization should map the process using a high-level flow diagram, identifying the various defects or known points of failure in the process and determining which is the highest priority or greatest leverage point to work on initially. A target for improvement should be determined. As previously mentioned, in most cases, 95% reliability is an appropriate target because it allows simpler designs.

The Design Work

The goal of the redesign work is to create processes that are clear, are easy to apply and understand, and can be routinely measured for reliable application by team members. There are three basic steps in designing an everyday practice for reliability:

1. Simplify and standardize to reach 80% reliability.

2. Apply an identification and mitigation step to achieve 95% reliability.

3. Identify defects and adjust the process to achieve continuous process improvement.

(*See* Figure 4-1 on page 36 for an illustration of the three-step design strategy and Figure 4-2 on page 40 for a checklist to help navigate the process.)

Step 1: Simplification and Standardization

The goal of step 1 is to achieve a level of reliability in terms of process output that is on the order of 80%–90%. Because many processes in health care involve multiple individuals

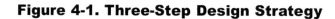

Figure 4-1. Three-Step Design Strategy

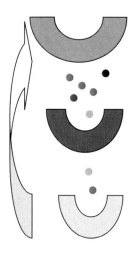

- Step 1: Simplification, standardization, and intent are used to help minimize the chance of process failure.

- Step 2: "Controls" are applied to help prevent error from occurring in the simplified process.

- Step 3: Errors that nevertheless occur are identified and interrupted before they cause harm.

Study the failures and redesign for exceptions if cost/benefit makes sense.

This figure shows the three steps to reliable design. The half circles reflect the levels of redundancy, and the dots illustrate that fewer defects are getting through. The arrow shows the need to have feedback to further improve.

Source: Doug Bonacum, Kaiser Permanente. Used with permission.

performing multiple steps in several ways—some of those steps being unnecessary—simplification and standardization can help achieve this first level of reliability.

Simplification is needed to reduce confusion and minimize waste. It is also needed to improve the inherent reliability of the system. At its core, simplification in process flow is about eliminating the unnecessary steps that increase the likelihood of error. As previously mentioned, the more steps involved in a process, the more likely there will be an error in that process. For example, if a process has one step that is reliably performed 95% of the time, there is a 95% chance that an individual will perform it correctly. Conversely, there is a 5% chance that the individual will perform it incorrectly. While this is pretty low risk for a single-step process, for each additional step in a process, the chances of error compound, so that by the time you have a 40-step process, there is only a 12% chance that all 40 steps in the process will be performed correctly. By simplifying the number and complexity of steps, you reduce the likelihood of error.

After unnecessary steps are eliminated, the next goal is to standardize the simplified process. Why is this important?

A single standardized process allows consistency and improves efficiency. Unfortunately, standardization is seldom done well in health care. Most clinical processes have a range of possible ways to accomplish a given task, and all these ways fall within the scope of acceptable medical practice. For years, clinicians have agreed that if there is a single standard based on good medical science, standardization is warranted. However, very few of these clinical opportunities exist.

The difficulty with allowing any acceptable process within the scope of practice is related to the lack of infrastructure to support multiple competing processes. For example, multiple approaches to potassium administration in the ICU can be problematic. The ability of the ICU to train all nurses and pharmacists in multiple approaches is limited. It involves training new employees in all of the approaches, following up on skills for current staff, coordinating which physicians desire which approaches, and following up on the efficacy of any one approach. By standardizing to one process, organizations can increase efficiency, reduce staff time, and ensure consistency. A single standardized care process allows the institutional expectation of training all the staff in the single protocol and following up on the efficacy of a single protocol.

One of the major benefits in standardizing care is that it helps to create a learning environment. The multiple methods approach makes the recognition of system defects difficult and the correction of defects in a particular protocol even more difficult. Standardization allows the detection of defects from the standardized care process and tracing the defect back to the cause. Each defect then becomes an opportunity to learn and improve the process.

Methods of Standardization. No standardized process can be expected to be successful if isolated experts try to develop the perfect protocol or standardized process without actually testing it in the clinical environment. Typically, a standardized protocol or care process is written by a group of experts in a nonexperiential setting, making an attempt to compromise and account for all possible objections and contingencies. The protocol or care process that results is, at worst, completely unworkable, or, at best, used by only a portion of the clinical staff, never spread to others, and has little ability to be sustained over time. With this type of experience, most clinicians and improvement staff have concluded that standardization of clinical processes is almost impossible.

The fault lies in the methodology of development and implementation, however, not in the fundamental concept of standardization. Successful implementation of a standardized process demands and expects local customization. This means that a given standard or protocol is essentially never "finished," but is always in a state of adjustment as providers find better ways to provide care. Following are some recommended steps to standardize a process:

• Step 1. Describe the current and ideal process. By observation, identification of problems, and drilling down for root causes of process failures, understand how the current process works. Describe the ideal process for management of the condition, using evidence from the literature, knowledge of the local environment, and any available local data. The description should include who, when, where, how, and with what.

• Step 2. Define and implement a practical measurement strategy. The measurement should be practical both for short-term testing and longer-term outcomes.

• Step 3. Write the protocol or care process. The first draft of the protocol or care process should be written by

several of the pertinent experts, taking a minimum of time, and utilizing out-of-organization examples of protocols, if necessary, just to get a start. The initial protocol or care process should be reflective of the few experts who will be willing to try the first version of the protocol on several patients within the next day or so. The protocol should be written in such a way that changes to the protocol or care process can be made within minutes. The goal for most organizations should be to include as few items as possible combined with good evidence.

• Step 4. Send out an early draft. Stakeholders should be encouraged to comment with short turnaround time limits to begin the buy-in process and improve the safety and robustness of the protocol.

• Step 5. Test an early draft of the protocol. The early draft of the protocol should be tested with a few patients. Immediately after these patients have been tested, the authors of the protocol should huddle with nurses and other staff who will be using the protocol to discuss what worked well and what needs to be changed. The information should immediately be incorporated into the protocol for the next series of tests.

• Step 6. Seek additional input from other interested participants. The initially tested and modified protocol should now be re-communicated with all other clinicians and staff who will eventually use the protocol, and further input requested. The input should then be used to remodel the protocol. The remodeled protocol should be tested and continually modified as needed.

• Step 7. Set expectations on use of the protocol. Expect either that the protocol will actually be used, or that the reason for opting out is communicated to the development team whenever a clinician decides not to use the protocol. This feedback information is crucial for remodeling and improving the protocol as necessary.

• Step 8. Assign a process or protocol owner. The ability to sustain a protocol is dependent on an owner. The owner of a protocol has several responsibilities, including being aware of any new literature that would impact the protocol, having available the compliance data regarding the use of the protocol, and having basic data regarding the reasons why the protocol is not being used, if applicable. No changes can be made to the protocol without consent and delegation of those changes from the process owner.

• Step 9. Remodel the protocol. Changes should be made to the protocol on the basis of the identified problems with the protocol or issues relating to the nonuse of the protocol. Modifications and improvements of the protocol should be an ongoing and continuous process. In essence, no protocol should ever be finished. The protocol should always be in the design mode.

Initial standardization of a care process will never be perfect, and the designers should expect failures. If an attempt is made in the initial design to deal with any and all probabilities that engage the clinical process, the initial protocol will become far too complicated. A complicated design is much more difficult to understand by the frontline staff that need to implement the protocol.

When the standardization process is inclusive and everyone has input, then acceptance and utilization increase. The process of testing, measuring, and improving the protocol also creates agreement between clinicians and provides certainty that the protocol is an improvement in care delivery.

As previously mentioned, the goal of step 1 is to achieve 80%–90% reliability. Your organization should have measures in place to gauge the reliability of the process. If it is not achieving 80%–90% reliability, then it should be redesigned and reworked to achieve the target reliability goal.

Step 2: Identification and Mitigation

Step 2 involves designing and implementing a process that "catches" those times when the step 1 process doesn't work and addressing the failures. Also known as the identification and mitigation step, it is critical to improving the reliability of a process. The second step allows for a less than perfect design in the standardization step, so you do not have to plan for every possible contingency in the first tier. For example, let's assume your organization's primary, standardized process for giving patients a pneumococcal vaccine is the nurse asking the patient during the final meeting before discharge whether he or she needs a pneumococcal vaccine and providing it when necessary. And let's assume that process works 80% of the time. Then to catch the 20% of patients not caught by the primary process you might implement a process in which visiting nurses who see the patient after discharge ask about the pneumococcal vaccine.

The goal of the second step is to catch 80% of the failures not caught in the primary process. Ultimately, if your second-step process catches 80% of the errors of the first-step process, your total system process will achieve 96% reliability.

The second step is really all about using human factors in a design to identify defects. (*See* Sidebar 4-1 on page 39.) A frequent approach is to use redundancy. Redundancies need to be carefully considered because they do represent a form of "waste" and should not be a complete reaudit. In general, they need to be independent of the original process used in the first step.

Within the second step you must set up a measurement tool to determine how often the step 2 process catches an error. A process rarely used will erode over time and not be dependable. A process used too frequently suggests a poorly designed first-tier standardization step and warrants some basic redesign.

Step 3: Failure Identification and Improvement

The effort in the third design step consists of two components. The first is the careful identification of failures that allow less than 80% reliability in the first two steps. The second is the careful creation of a direct link between these defects and a proposed redesign. All designs need a measurement of defects. Understanding why initial designs fail, and using the information about failures to redesign, is an essential part of reliability work. These defects provide the learning necessary to take the design to the desired level of reliability. The causes of the observed defects need to be prioritized, and then the highest-priority defects used for redesigning either the first or second tier. For this to occur, both components of the third tier need to be in place. The feedback loop to the design should be deliberate and swift to ensure rapid redesign. Failures in this phase of reliable design may be detected through tools such as routine electronic surveillance of data banks or manual audits of charts. For example, when a patient is not vaccinated either prior to discharge or during a nurse visit, the process is designed so that the surveillance system detects the issue, flags it for follow-up, and prompts consideration for redesign, as appropriate.

By performing a series of "small tests of change" and measuring their impact, a team can rapidly move from the "setup" phase of reliable design, all the way through step 3. A small test of change is nothing more than an idea that is tried on a small scale to see if it will result in an improvement. If the test is successful, it can be expanded to larger and larger sample sizes until there is confidence that the change should be adopted more widely.[5] For example, if testing a new method in a small office practice to validate that a specimen

---

Sidebar 4-1. Human Factors Engineering Strategies

Human factors engineering strategies to use in redesigning processes include the following:

- Avoid reliance on memory. This may involve designing processes to involve checklists, forced reminders, mnemonic devices, and so forth.

- Use constraints/forcing functions. These are functions that make it easy to do the right thing and hard to do the wrong thing. For example, in a computerized provider order entry system a constraint may be a notice that pops up on-screen when you enter an incorrect dose of medication. A forcing function in such a system may not allow you to proceed to the next screen without first performing a certain task, such as verifying allergies.

- Use protocols and checklists to generate standard care and, as previously mentioned, ensure that a procedure is performed consistently because the checklist detects inadvertent omission without relying on human memory.

- Decrease "look-alikes" and "sound-alikes." When two things look alike, it is easy to mistake one for the other. Consider the soda aisle of a grocery store. The brand-name cola is often placed next to a generic that has the same color label and font style. The differences between the labels are subtle, and when consumers are distracted or in a hurry, they may mistake one for the other. The same applies in health care with medications, supplies, equipment, and so forth. By reducing look-alikes, organizations can ensure that individuals will correctly identify the right product even when in a hurry, distracted, fatigued, or stressed. Within its National Patient Safety Goals, The Joint Commission requires organizations to limit look-alike medications to improve the reliability of medication delivery. In addition, The Joint Commission requires organizations to label all medications, medication containers (for example, syringes, medicine cups, basins), or other solutions on and off the sterile field to ensure accurate identification of medication and prevent medication error.

- Reduce the number of handoffs. The more times a patient is handed off to another provider, the more times important information about that patient can be lost. By limiting handoffs, you can limit the opportunity for error. Whenever handoffs are necessary, they should be structured so that consistent and comprehensive communication takes place every time. More about communication during handoffs can be found in Chapter 6.

- Automate carefully. As discussed in Chapter 10, although technology offers significant potential for improvement in quality, safety, and efficiency, the risk of technology-associated accidents looms large. Before implementing automation and technology, make sure that the process you are automating is effective, that the technology will ensure the consistent functioning of the process, and that the technology will not lead to work-arounds or other new sources of error. Limited pilot projects that are carefully tracked can prevent major technology-induced problems.

- Take advantage of habits and patterns. If a new process works within the current habits and patterns of the participants in the process, they are more likely to embrace the new process and follow it. People inherently do not like change, so if a process can use components of an existing process it can prove to be more beneficial.

---

container is appropriately labeled, the change might be tried with one physician and one medical assistant in one office with one patient. With an acceptable outcome for, say, a total of 10 consecutive patients, the test might then be expanded to cover two clinical teams. If the outcomes are similar, a plan to spread the practice to the remaining three physicians in the office may be developed. After the process is part of routine operations and spread as appropriate, future failures can be studied, and redesign implemented if it makes sense from a cost/benefit perspective.

ADDRESSING THE CULTURAL ASPECTS OF RELIABILITY

As mentioned in Chapter 1, designing reliable processes is only one step in becoming a high-reliability organization. Your organization must address the cultural component as well. A clear example of the need to address culture when designing for reliability is the often doubted efficacy of bar coding, a technology that from an engineering and reliable process perspective is a "no brainer." The issue with bar coding in many organizations, however, may be more about the organization's culture, patient safety values, how the technology is socialized in the organization, and how leaders listen and respond to staff members who are having trouble using it safely.

Likewise, the ongoing debate about the efficacy of rapid response teams appears to be one grounded in culture as well. If the concept of the rapid response team is not appropriately introduced in an organization, if the culture is not "just" nor one where it's safe to speak up, and if the organization doesn't place a high value on continuous learning from both the appropriate use of and failure to use the system, rapid response teams might be another great safety idea that falls short in execution.

Figure 4-2. Reliable Design Checklist

Step 1: Standardization, Simplification, and Intent
Standardization and simplification of process
- "What" should be done? (based on good medical evidence).
- "How" can that be done? (does not need medical evidence but systems knowledge).

Ensure that each step is necessary: reducing # of steps can reduce error.
Initial standardized protocols: small-time investment by experts
Customization initially: required and encouraged
Changes are possible when generally accepted, but monitored.
Design the process so you can learn from each defect.
Leadership must drive expectation of standardization.
Model shifts from "opt in" to "opt out"
Designated process owner
Reach 80%–90% compliance before next step.

Step 2: Apply Controls
Decision aids and reminders built into the system
- Use hierarchy of controls (mitigate–facilitate–eliminate).

Teamwork and communication tools used
Desired action is the default (based on evidence).
Building process into scheduled steps (for example, daily rounds)
Take advantage of habits and patterns (for example, change-of-shift report).
Aim is to reach 90% to 95% before next step is designed.

Step 3: Identification and Mitigation
Through the use of redundancies, failures that occur are identified and mitigated (before they cause harm) to go as far beyond 95% reliability as feasible.
Make sure you have a way to count how many times the redundancy is needed to stop harm (for example, if needed more than 5%–10% of the time, revisit the design).

Ongoing Process Improvement
Measure critical *failures*.
If you are going to pursue, this is where "customization" occurs—that is, a different process may be needed for outliers.
This should be used to redesign the process when appropriate (> 10% failure).

This figure offers a checklist that organizations can use to help navigate the reliable design process.
Source: Institute for Healthcare Improvement. Used with permission.

Ensuring effective teamwork and communication, developing a just culture and accountability system, and examining mistakes in order to learn from them are just some of the concepts that must be in place to achieve a culture of reliability. Another piece is to develop an organizational intolerance for ambiguity and work-arounds. Spear compares and contrasts the health care system of the United States with the Toyota Production System,[6] noting that health care workers work around ambiguities, meeting patients' immediate needs but not resolving the ambiguities themselves. As a result, people confront the same problem, every day, for years, manifested as inefficiencies and irritations—and, occasionally, as catastrophes. Unless everyone is completely clear about the tasks that must be done, exactly who should be doing them, and just how they should be performed, Spear notes, the potential for error will always be high.

PURSUING RISK RESILIENCE

The journey to high reliability continues with the development of resilience. *Resilience* is the ability to manage situations that arise when all contingencies have been addressed and failure still occurs.

Organizations must understand that even with 95% or greater reliability and the best-designed systems, defects will still occur. Processes will fail in novel ways that cannot always be predicted. The success of an organization in achieving high reliability will depend on its ability to detect, address, or contain failures, and bounce back.

Hollnagel describes three models of risk resilience[7]: The first is a simple linear model that invokes a domino scenario in which an initiating event starts an unstoppable cascade. The second is a complex linear model (such as that described by Reason's Swiss Cheese Model of Accident Causation[8]) with latent defects and the possibility of conditional prediction (*see* page 29 in Chapter 3). For example, if you know and correct the latent defects, you can prevent future events. Finally, the nonlinear or systemic model is applicable when concurrences of multiple factors, some of which may have no apparent prior relationship, cause the event.

Hollnagel says, "Accepting a specific model does not only have consequences for how accidents are understood, but also for how resilience is seen. In a simple linear model, resilience is the same as being impervious to specific causes; using the domino analogy, the pieces either cannot fall or are so far apart that the fall of one cannot affect its neighbours. In a complex linear model, resilience is the ability to maintain effective barriers that can withstand the impact of harmful agents and the erosion that is the result of latent conditions. . . . In contrast to that, a systemic model adopts a functional point of view in which resilience is an organisation's ability efficiently to adjust to harmful influences rather than to shun or resist them."[6(p. 14)]

Perhaps the best design advice that comes from Hollnagel's analysis of risk resilience models is as follows:

1. Components of a process and their interrelationship with each other must be made as reliable as possible.

2. Barriers or safeguards must be built into processes to reduce the risk of even the most reliable components failing.

3. The processes and people within an organization must be able to flex and respond to hazards and failures that nevertheless occur

As mentioned previously, processes have to be made reliable or the organization will face so many defects that staff members will spend most of their time addressing the many failures in poorly designed processes. After processes are made reliable, the staff can then move to develop an approach to resilience that can be implemented when rare defects occur.

To develop resilience, an organization must have knowledge about the technology in place, the system in question, the workers, and the materials used. An example of technol-ogy may be the sensitivity and specificity of the alerts that appear when prescribing a medication. An example of workers may be the skills and capacity of workers to address sudden changes in volume.

Resilient organizations both learn from their failures and proactively perform under a variety of simulated conditions so they are adequately prepared to manage the unexpected. Organizations such as Cincinnati Children's Hospital Medical Center are furthering their resiliency by developing profound situational awareness through formalized routines and structures that are aimed at predicting difficulties, taking action to mitigate the risk of occurrence before the prediction becomes a reality, and then being fully prepared if an event should nevertheless occur.[9] For example, a daily (Monday–Friday) 20-minute housewide safety brief represents one such routine. During the daily safety brief, which key leaders from across the medical center attend, statistics regarding worker and patient safety are shared. Each department reports on quality and safety issues that have occurred since the last brief (the "look-back") and also "looks ahead" to what it expects or can reasonably predict to happen in the next 24 hours. The daily safety brief also provides an opportunity to follow up on issues previously identified that have not yet been resolved. Cincinnati Children's has found that this process helps foster accountability, increase situational awareness, and improve risk resilience.

Macrae describes five key process dimensions that frame the concept of risk resilience in the airline industry.[10] Comparable simple examples of how these defenses have been used in health care safety design have been added to his classifications:

1. Processes (defenses) are in place that maintain defenses against possible failures in case they occur. This means that even if there is little chance of an event occurring, the defense is still operational.

Health Care Example: Administration of penicillin to a patient who has no known allergy to penicillin and has taken the antibiotic previously. The nurse would be trained and procedures would be developed whereby all the symptoms of an allergic reaction would be monitored just as one would do with a patient of questionable allergic history. The defenses are maintained in case the reaction occurs.

2. Processes (defenses) are in place that provide numerous means to catch failures for any operational situation.

Designs would be such that multiple methods would exist to catch failures in care.

Health Care Example: Use of two identifiers for blood drawing in the laboratory. The patient name and birthday are two common identifiers required at each blood draw. In this situation, if two John Smiths are having blood drawn, the addition of the birth date helps confirm the correct patient.

3. Processes (defenses) are in place that add layers of additional defenses beyond any that are actually called upon to catch a failure.

Health Care Example: The process related to type matching, crossmatching, and the eventual transfusion of blood. The blood draw team uses the two identifiers, as described, and a specific blood transfusion number is generated. After the blood is in the transfusion department, another individual conducts another verification. Before the transfusion itself, the blood transfusion number, along with the two identifiers, is used by the person who delivers the blood and the nurse administering the blood to ensure the correct person and the correct blood.

4. Processes (defenses) are in place working to reduce and avoid the occurrence of failure in the first place.

Health Care Example: The design of quiet areas in the hospital so shift-to-shift exchange of information can occur without interruptions.

5. Processes (defenses) are in place that ensure a systematic organizational approach to safety.

Health Care Example: A nonsystematic approach would be a surgeon who is highly vigilant regarding his method for identifying the correct side of surgery. Because of his vigilance and hard work, his patients have the correct side of surgery marked by him as outpatients and then they sign the site. He has had no near misses or events related to wrong-side surgery in his 40-year career. Unfortunately, he performs surgical marking differently from all the other sur-

geons in the hospital. His safety record is based on a fortuitous skill set but does not represent an organizational approach to the problem of wrong-side surgery.

Resiliency is an adaptive response to a situation, which some may see as being in conflict with building reliable processes. According to this view, if the goal of reliability is to implement standardized process, permitting an adaptive response may mean that workers will not use the standardized process. Resiliency requires prediction, adaptability, flexibility, and innovation. Yet, in fact, it is this adaptability that allows an organization to capture those defects that are not captured by the reliable processes that are built for situations that can be predicted and managed with a standardized approach.

REFERENCES

1. Berwick D, Nolan T. High reliability health care. Paper presented at the Institute for Healthcare Improvement's 15th Annual Forum on Quality Improvement in Health Care, New Orleans, Dec 2003.
2. McGlynn EA, et al. The quality of health care delivered to adults in the United States. *N Engl J Med.* 2003 Jun 26;348(26):2635–2645.
3. Reinertsen JL. Zen and the art of physician autonomy maintenance. *Ann Intern Med.* 2003 Jun 17;138(12):992–995.
4. Vaughan D. *The Challenger Launch Decision: Risky Technology, Culture, and Deviance at NASA.* Chicago: University of Chicago Press, 1996.
5. Langley GJ, et al. *The Improvement Guide: A Practical Guide to Enhancing Organizational Performance,* 2nd ed. San Francisco: Jossey-Bass, 2009.
6. Spear SJ. Fixing healthcare from the inside: Teaching residents to heal broken delivery processes as they heal sick patients. *Acad Med.* 2006;81(10 Suppl):S144–149.
7. Hollnagel E. Resilience: The challenge of the unstable. In Hollnagel E., Woods DD, Leveson N, editors: *Resilience Engineering: Concepts and Precepts.* Aldershot, UK: Ashgate Publishing, 2006, 9–17.
8. Reason J. Human error: Models and management. *BMJ.* 2000 Mar 18;320(7237):768–770.
9. Cincinnati Children's Hospital Medical Center. HRO Leadership Methods: Daily Safety Brief. Video. Sep 22, 2011. Accessed Oct 31, 2012. http://seraph.cchmc.org/mediasiteex/Viewer/?peid=50a48b3628c047538923e61e9e74f893.
10. Macrae CJ. Assuring Organizational Risk Resilience: Assessing, Managing and Learning from Flight Safety Incident Reports (PhD thesis). University of East Anglia, Dec 2005.

Chapter Five

SYSTEMATIC FLOW OF INFORMATION: THE EVOLUTION OF WALKROUNDS

Allan Frankel, MD; Sarah Pratt, MPH

One of the primary tenets of this book is that leaders should foster an environment in which errors, near misses, risks, and problems are discussed openly and honestly, and then acted on. To do this, organizations must have a systematic flow of information from frontline staff to organization leadership and back again. This helps ensure a reliable system in which problems and risks are consistently identified; identified issues are analyzed; staff concerns are responded to; and risks are addressed in such a way that experience facilitates prevention, identification, or mitigation of future errors. An organization that has a systematic flow of information takes a significant step toward high reliability and enhances its patient safety and performance.

Critical elements involved in systemizing the flow of information are as follows:

• Easy-to-use methods of capturing information about problems or issues

• Leadership support of and active participation in these methods

• A consistently reinforced message to staff that speaking up or reporting concerns and events is an esteemed action that may be done safely. A systematic flow of information is predicated on a robust, easily understandable accountability system in which staff members know when they will be held accountable for safety and reliability failures and when the organization will hold accountable the systems that support the provision of health care in the organization. As discussed in Chapter 3, organizations must assess accountability consistently to ensure that the staff knows how the organization will respond to problems or errors.

• A mechanism for organizing and ranking the information collected. Most organizations don't have the time

and funds to fix every problem that staff members encounter. By prioritizing, organizations can determine, out of the 100 problems identified, which 5 are the most important to fix right away. One effective method for ranking information is to consider the severity of the issue and multiply it by how many times that issue occurs. Issues that are high severity and high frequency should go to the top of the list.[1] Organizations may also consider fixing issues that are low severity but high frequency, as these are the little irritations that staff face every day. High-severity, low-frequency events may also be important to address, depending on the nature of the problem and the likelihood of occurrence.

• An owner for the information gathering, analysis, and response process. Recently, organizations are combining quality and safety and risk departments to support this effort.

• Prompt acknowledgement of reports. Even if you cannot fix a problem right away, it is important to acknowledge the report and outline what the next steps are in addressing it.

• Regular and comprehensive communication about issue resolution. When an issue is resolved, you must communicate to everyone about the nature of the problem and how it was fixed. It's important for staff members to see action as a result of their speaking up or reporting. If they believe that when they do so nothing will be done about it, they will stop reporting.

This chapter focuses on WalkRounds, introduced as *Leadership* (or *Executive*) WalkRounds (and also known as *walk-rounds*), which represents one way of establishing a systematic flow of information. In WalkRounds, management and frontline staff engage in a structured, two-way conversation about safety, and data from that conversation are captured, analyzed, prioritized, and addressed.[2] On the whole, the WalkRounds process is designed to do the following:

- Show that senior leaders are promoting patient safety efforts.

- Hear the concerns of frontline providers. Through WalkRounds, leaders get to directly interact with staff, learn the unfiltered truth about issues, and directly influence the tone of the culture.

- Increase mutual understanding between senior leaders and frontline staff about patient safety issues.

- Support appropriate accountability.

- Foster a culture of teamwork and continuous learning.

- Allocate resources to areas of greatest risk.

WalkRounds was conceptualized initially in 1999 as an effort to engage leaders in patient safety.[2,3] Since then, it has been increasingly recognized and appreciated that health care leaders' full engagement in patient safety efforts is a powerful force in cultural change toward achieving reliable care.[4,5] The WalkRounds concept remains useful, even as it has evolved in response to the growing understanding of safety and reliability.

The idea of WalkRounds took hold in response to the Institute of Medicine's report *To Err Is Human*[6] as quality and patient safety staff sought a way to engage senior hospital leaders in safety work. They perceived that leaders needed to carry the banner of safety in their institutions as a mechanism to engage providers in a discussion about errors and improving the reliability of care. Meanwhile, the Institute for Healthcare Improvement's (IHI) patient safety faculty had learned from their experience with year-long patient safety collaboratives that hospital improvement teams were more likely to succeed if hospital leaders were actively engaged in safety efforts. Most hospital leaders knew little about human factors, a just culture,[7,8] or redesign of clinical systems for clinical reliability,[9] let alone focus on patient safety and medical errors in their corporate strategy. When IHI's 1999 "Quantum Leaps" Patient Safety collaborative required participating leaders to engage in a prescriptive patient safety program called WalkRounds, we filled a void with a nascent but logical management tool. Soon after, the WalkRounds concept spread, and one of the first studies showed that the leader-worker conversation during WalkRounds changed perceptions about safety and increased the likeli-

hood that improvement for the better might occur.[10] Other published studies, such as Ghandi et al.,[11] have shown that WalkRounds increased employees' willingness to speak about their concerns and report safety issues, reflecting the "psychological safety" that is critical in a safety culture (*see* Chapter 6).

In 2000 the president of Boston's Brigham and Women's Hospital (BWH), Jeff Otten, agreed to pilot a WalkRounds program to proactively identify patient safety risks and promote a culture of safety. Otten came from the world of health care finance but had published an article earlier in his career about rounding to talk to patients,[12] so the idea of extending those rounds to patient safety appealed to him. BWH began carefully orchestrated weekly WalkRounds, and within six months, the BWH patient safety director and manager, each had enough experience with the process to refine it, and with BWH leadership permission, to make it permanent. The evolution of WalkRounds at BWH is described in Sidebar 5-1 (page 45).

When WalkRounds was first conceived, we instructed senior leaders to engage in a discussion with their frontline personnel about safety and then engage everyone in improvement efforts to address the issues. In the first step, senior leaders went to the clinical units and ask providers (1) how patients might get hurt as a result of delivering care, (2) for specific examples of patient harm, and (3) what barriers existed to delivering safe care. These were then unusual questions for leaders to ask. The second part of WalkRounds required that the conversations be carefully documented and then the issues discussed and analyzed, and solutions identified and acted on. A detailed "Guide to Conduct WalkRounds" is provided on pages 46–51.

Early experience indicated that if leaders and safety personnel focused on the first part of WalkRounds—the unit-based discussion—but failed to rapidly advance to an effective second step of resolving issues, then leaders quickly tired of the rounds. Repeatedly hearing about the same problems was frustrating and detracted from the primary purpose of WalkRounds, which was to engage with frontline providers to empower them to make changes and improvements. Performing even a few rounds generated a long list of issues, some amenable to easy solutions, others emblematic of everything that is complex in health care and difficult to fix. In the hospitals that did not appreciate the necessity of

Sidebar 5-1. The Evolution of WalkRounds at Brigham and Women's Hospital

Allen Kachalia, MD, JD; Lisa Rubino; Erin Graydon Baker, MS, RRT

Executive WalkRounds continues to be a valuable component of Patient Safety efforts at Brigham and Women's Hospital (BWH). The primary focus has not changed, but the program has evolved during the past decade.

WalkRounds Team Members

When BWH first launched Executive WalkRounds, the sessions included one senior executive (the CEO, chief operating officer, chief medical officer, or chief nursing officer), the director of patient safety, the patient safety manager, the medication safety officer, and a scribe. The sessions also included site-specific personal such as the vice president, nurse director, nurse–in-charge, department manager, and medical director. As the sessions grew in popularity, additional members were added to the core group, including risk management, biomedical engineering, the chief information officer (once a month), and information system managers.

For each session, we visit one discrete clinical area or unit in the hospital for the full hour session. This scheduling process allows us to visit each inpatient area about once every two years and each ambulatory area once every three to four years. Today, the chief quality officer and chief financial officer are also part of the senior-executive rotation.

WalkRounds Preparation

We schedule every WalkRounds session a year in advance to ensure participation from our senior executives, each of whom leads four WalkRounds per year. When we launched WalkRounds, we would send a set of 12 to 15 sample questions to the clinical unit's leadership a few days before the session. The sample questions were sent to help participants prepare for the session. Before each WalkRounds session, the patient safety team reviews comments and action items from previous WalkRounds and the safety events reported by that unit to helps the facilitator spark conversation. In addition, reviewing the safety event reports has several benefits: The unit realizes that someone actually reviews the safety reports they file, and it allows the staff to give us more information on the events and how we can help.

WalkRounds Session

We begin each session with an introduction, led by the patient safety team. This introduction offers the opportunity for the senior leadership to meet the staff and for the team to explain the WalkRounds process. Setting the stage at the beginning of the WalkRounds allows us to make it clear that the intent of the session is to learn which systems put our patients at risk for harm; they are not held for placing blame or judgment. The scribe records the comments and sends the highlights to participants about a week after the WalkRounds.

Post-WalkRounds

After the WalkRounds, the patient safety team reviews all staff comments from the session and develops draft action items. These action items are then reviewed with the appropriate service vice president, who subsequently assigns the action items to the appropriate subject matter expert for resolution. For example, any action item associated with our computer systems is referred to one of the information systems supervisors. The patient safety team tracks the action items until they are resolved.

After the action items from each WalkRounds are resolved, the patient safety team updates all participants, including the frontline staff and senior leaders, of the "fixes" via e-mail. BWH has been trending and reporting the percentage of WalkRounds action items completed within six months, with a goal of at least 75% for closing actions within that period. For example, as of February 2010, 74.5% of action items were closed within six months, increasing to 94.2% by January 2011.

Lessons Learned and Future WalkRounds Enhancements

Success of the WalkRounds relies on the communication of WalkRounds notes, action items, and systems fixes to frontline staff after each session. We send follow-up to all WalkRounds participants that highlight the changes resulting from their comments. Along the way, we have found that large groups hindered our ability to conduct WalkRounds directly on the unit department without interfering with patient care. Large groups, particularly when many senior leaders are involved, may also be intimidating to frontline staff and impede the open sharing of staff's safety concerns. Therefore, at the start of 2011, we changed the WalkRounds attendance in an effort to improve the direct and candid conversations with frontline staff. We pared the group down from a potential of 15 or more attendees, to a total of 5 to 8. Now, in addition to a senior executive, the core group of participants consists of the patient safety manager, the area's vice president, the executive nursing director or the physician director, unit/department-level manager, the medication safety officer, and the scribe.

In an effort to reach more frontline staff, we now visit two clinical locations or units on every WalkRounds. Aside from increasing staff exposure to the senior executives, this change allows us to visit more areas annually. Finally, we no longer send a list of sample questions to the unit/department's leader so as not to encourage staff to "prepare" answers before the session. Past experiences had shown that WalkRounds work best when staff have not preselected issues to discuss. Since implementation of this new process, WalkRounds seem more effective and allow for more candid conversations with staff.

We are enhancing our current follow-up process to send routine reminders to leadership of open items. This will hopefully allow us to "close" action items faster and communicate with frontline staff in a more timely fashion. In addition, a monthly Patient Safety Executive Committee now helps expedite follow-up of patient safety events, regardless of how they are reported or identified. At the committee meetings, we routinely review the larger and more complicated safety concerns raised at WalkRounds. This routine review ensures not only that hospital leadership is aware of the concerns identified on WalkRounds but that the concerns are tracked until resolved.

Source: Brigham and Women's Hospital, Boston. Used with permission.

rigorous follow-up, the WalkRounds process, half implemented, tended to wither.

WalkRounds, fully implemented, was a different story. Aside from providing leaders with a prescribed technique to engage in patient safety, it described a mechanism for quality and safety departments to study adverse event and near-miss data, and then act on that information to improve. Those who systematically tackled the issues found the program useful on a few fronts. Hospital leaders learned a great deal, safety issues were tackled more effectively, and frontline providers did engage, repeatedly summing up the experience with a powerfully motivating sentiment, "We feel like we're being heard."

Organizations across the world are still using the WalkRounds program as a mechanism to engage senior leaders in efforts to improve the reliability of care in their organizations. Two additional organizations now describe their WalkRounds experiences. The South West region of the National Health Service (NHS) of England initiated WalkRounds as part of a patient safety collaborative and has sustained the activity, with efforts to spread the program to other care providers (*see* Sidebar 5-2, page 47). Sunnybrook Health Center (Toronto) has made numerous adaptations to the WalkRounds program since its initial implementation in 2004 (*see* Sidebar 5-3, pages 48–49).

REFLECTIONS

The great strength of WalkRounds, in its original design, is that senior leaders engage in discussions about safety and reliability and ensure that the banner of safety is carried high. Its potential drawback is that it spreads the attention of a few leaders across an entire organization, thereby thinning out the impact and generating a long list of not always solvable problems.

The advantage of assigning a leader to one unit for a defined period of time is that it generates a close(r) relationship between that leader and the unit's frontline providers. However, the risk is that the effort concentrates on only one or a small number of units, limiting the overall organizational impact of leadership engagement. In addition, the focus may be on one aspect of care and not elicit from providers their frustrations and concerns about a broader array of safety issues.

The questions posed during WalkRounds about harm to patients are now more frequently asked, although leaders are still learning how to effectively conduct the conversa-

tions. For example, whereas some organizations have found that providing a list of the questions ahead of time was helpful, others have preferred to have spontaneous conversations. Other factors, such as leadership's skill in directing the conversation, may play a more significant role. Although WalkRounds are no longer as critical as they once were in making providers aware of safety, they remain useful in engaging and teaching leaders, improving the way we improve, and ultimately in delivering safer and more reliable care.

A GUIDE TO CONDUCT WALKROUNDS*

The WalkRounds process is fairly straightforward and includes the following seven steps:

1. Preparation. This step involves garnering commitment and regular participation by leadership, securing dedicated resources from quality and safety departments, and clearly defining the process, scheduling, and feedback mechanisms for the rest of the organization.

2. Scheduling. To be effective, organizations should consider setting WalkRounds months in advance and accommodate schedules of executive team members, supporting patient safety staff, and other participants. Canceling these scheduled rounds should be strongly discouraged, with agreement that rather than ever canceling, leaders commit to rescheduling within a short time frame.

3. Conducting WalkRounds. A first step is to decide where to conduct the sessions. WalkRounds take about an hour to complete and can occur at any site in the organization where employees or clinicians are directly involved in patient care or support the process, including all hospital floors, radiology, emergency rooms, pharmacies, ambulatory settings, and outpatient offices. WalkRounds have also been done in the hospital billing office, in central sterilization units, in transportation departments, and on floors dedicated to hospital information technology systems. When choosing a site, you may want to consider starting with those units in which the safety climate score—of the safety culture survey discussed in Chapter 2—is less than 60. This indicates an area in which a strong rapport between leadership and frontline staff could be very beneficial.

When conducting the WalkRounds, you may hold the discussion on the floor or department in an open area

---

* Adapted from Frankel A, Grillo S, Pittman M. *Patient Safety Leadership WalkRounds™ Guide*. Cambridge, MA: Institute for Healthcare Improvement, 2004.

Sidebar 5-2. Sustaining and Spreading WalkRounds

Peter Cavanagh, MB BChir, NHS South West, England

The concept of Patient Safety WalkRounds was introduced to the South West region of the National Health Service (NHS) of England in 2007, when 4 of its 18 acute care hospitals took part in the Safer Patients Initiative (SPI) collaborative supported by the Institute for Healthcare Improvement (IHI).[1] Following the success of this initiative, since 2008 the South West has expanded a patient safety collaborative across its 18 acute care, 8 mental health care, and 13 community health care providers. WalkRounds, identified as one of the keys to success in the initial SPI work, are now an integral part of the patient safety collaborative in all health care settings. However most of the knowledge we have about WalkRounds is based on our experience in acute care.

Most of the organizations have kept to the original format, as developed through SPI and shared in a how-to guide produced as part of the national Patient Safety First campaign of England.[2,3] In the standard format, all executive directors are provided a comprehensive timetable of visits, which is intended to cover the entire organization on at least an annual basis.

Visiting Teams
In first implementing WalkRounds, executives often pair up, a clinical executive joining with a nonclinical executive. At most of the organizations, the visiting team is then composed of one executive and a patient safety officer. Some of the larger organizations include others, such as divisional director, on the teams. None of the organizations include a patient directly in the visit, although some organizations take the opportunity to visit and speak to a patient or patients in the unit—usually at the end of the visit. One organization asks that a patient story be brought back and shared from all visits to a clinical area.

At one organization, some of their WalkRounds involve following a particular issue through from department to department. For example, for the issue of failure to make a timely transfer of patients from the operating room (OR) back to the wards because of lack of bed availability, a team first visited the OR and then visited the ward that was causing a particular problem. The team then found that the ward was waiting for pharmacy to dispense To-Take-Out's before they could discharge patients. The team then went to pharmacy in an effort to understand why the work wasn't "flowing."

Measures
All of the organizations in the WalkRounds program are encouraged to deliver on two measures: (1) number of WalkRounds performed per month and the number of completed actions and (2) number of actions identified through WalkRounds that are completed.

The limitations of these metrics are understood. Recording the number of WalkRounds does not reflect any measure of the quality of the dialogue during a visit. Some of the organizations performing less well on WalkRounds attempt to combine the visits to the clinical areas with other activities, such as communicating non–patient safety-related information to frontline staff. In addition, some organizations carry out the visits with no agreed-on follow-up actions, whereas others generate too many follow-up actions for the organizations to be able to address (we recommend no more than three per visit).

Progress
One of the keys to success is the CEO's promotion of WalkRounds as a high-value activity, as reflected, for example, in its integration into the executive team's strategic program, with weekly reporting back on the key issues and follow-up actions. In addition, the executive team should share information about the program with the organization's operational management, as is done at one organization at its weekly regular service-head meetings. Leaders need to view their participation in WalkRounds as a key part of their role and understand the learning opportunity it offers to them and the board. There needs to be a well-organized timetable of visits and a database that can track the actions and their completion. And, finally, there needs to be a timely feedback loop to the frontline staff to ensure that they understand that their views are listened to and addressed.

Spread of the WalkRounds to the mental health organizations has started with inpatient facilities. The development of WalkRounds in the community setting has been more challenging, primarily because of geographic issues. One of the community health care providers, which oversees 13 small community hospitals, has developed a structured program of visits to all sites by members of its executive team. However, to make these time-efficient (the traveling time can be more than two hours), they have combined the visit with other activities, such as staff meetings.

References
1. Health Foundation. *Learning Report: Safer Patients Initiative*. London: Health Foundation, Feb 2011. Accessed Oct 21, 2012. http://www.health.org.uk/publications/safer-patients-initiative.
2. Patient Safety First. About Patient Safety First. Accessed Oct 31, 2012. http://www.patientsafetyfirst.nhs.uk/Content.aspx?path=/About-the-campaign/.
3. *Patient Safety First. Patient Safety First 2008 to 2010: The Campaign Review*. London: Patient Safety First, Mar 2011. Accessed Oct 21, 2012. http://www.patientsafetyfirst.nhs.uk/ashx/Asset.ashx?path=Patient%20Safety%20First%20-%20the%20campaign%20review.pdf.

Source: NHS South West, England. Used with permission.

Sidebar 5-3. WalkArounds at Sunnybrook Health Sciences Centre

Guna Budrevics, CCHSA(A),CPHQ

WalkArounds at Sunnybrook Health Sciences Centre were initiated in 2004 by Sunnybrook's patient safety service. An academic and research centre located in Toronto, with 1,212 beds, more than 10,000 employees and volunteers, Sunnybrook specializes in cancer, cardiac, high-risk obstetrics, and trauma care. WalkArounds are consistent with our overall patient safety efforts, which are intended to promote a culture of safety through reliable design of systems and measurement.

The WalkArounds Process

Every two weeks, a senior leader conducts a 90-minute dialogue with multidisciplinary representatives from a unit. Given the ratio of units in the organization and available senior leaders, each senior leader conducts two to three WalkArounds a year. Questions are precirculated to the unit, along with a summary of recent safety reports. These documents serve as cues to both the leader and participants in focusing the discussion on harms, reporting culture, risks, and frequency of events.

As the participants discuss their unit's patient safety concerns, the facilitator records the issues on flip charts, and at the end of the session, the team collectively ranks and selects three priority issues for the senior leader to escalate for resolution with the appropriate personnel within the organization. The unit dialogue is frequently followed by a tour of the area to better visualize some of the concerns, and photos are taken to assist the team with subsequent communication. All issues are entered into a database to support the tracking of organizationwide patient safety themes, along with the progress and completion of priority issues. The automated process from identification through to resolution is a critical component of WalkArounds. Reminders for follow-up are sent to leaders until a solution is agreed upon by the senior leader and the unit manager, who is expected to share the outcomes with their staff. This demonstrates to stakeholders the shared accountability and leadership necessary to fully address patient safety concerns and improvements.

Accountability for Outcomes

Although the WalkArounds process is coordinated through the Department of Quality and Patient Safety, all participants play a significant role in the process. Ultimately, each senior leader is accountable for initiating a response to priority issues identified in each visit, as well as conducting a focused and balanced conversation about the local safety culture. Unit-based leaders contribute by providing insight into the unit's microculture and assist in facilitating solutions to the actionable items. The participants come prepared to share their concerns: Some teams consult with all staff before the WalkAround to ensure balanced representation of the unit's patient safety concerns. A member of the Patient Safety Leadership Team—a group of risk management, patient safety, and performance improvement

professionals—acts as the coordinating and facilitating resource for WalkArounds.

The director of Quality and Patient Safety meets quarterly with senior leadership to review progress on outstanding priority items and review the trends seen in the overall findings. This provides management with a valuable organizationwide scan of current frontline concerns, as well as contextual data about how effectively patient safety improvements are being translated at the bedside.

Adaptations

We have made a series of adaptations to the original WalkArounds model,[1] including data management, issue classification, board involvement, orientation, and identification and description of issues.

Data management. Our initial attempts at managing the findings, actions, and reports via spreadsheets were eclipsed within a few years due to volume. We partnered with a risk management software vendor, who worked with us in 2008 to adapt an application that suited our reporting and communication needs. We are now able to inform and manage the entire process more effectively and improve turnaround times for the completion of priority items.

Issue classification. We significantly condensed a list of categories of contributing factors[2] to simplify input into the database. We have been able to sustain the integrity of the 8 classifications (of the 29 original classifications) selected—Environmental, Teamwork/Communication, Formal Rules & Policies, Safeguards, Organizational, Patient, Individual, and Other.

Board involvement. In 2008 we invited interested board members to observe how WalkArounds unfold. In addition to attending the WalkAround, each board member was apprised of the actions and resolution of the priority issues.

Orientation. All senior-level participants (senior leaders new to the organization and board participants) attend a short orientation to understand the value of WalkArounds as a proactive patient safety tool. The package includes speakers' notes, suggested facilitation questions, a WalkArounds process map, and outlines of roles and responsibilities.

Identification and description of issues. As we become better at conducting WalkArounds, we also become more adept at describing the conditions to be addressed. Asking participants how frequently a process failure/incident occurs, for example, helps to shape the conversation about needed actions and resolution. Similarly, as the organization continues to improve and integrates more patient safety best practices, we continue to shape and modify the scripts and phrasing to reflect new behavioral targets.

Measurement

The key metrics are the number of issues (priority and nonpriority) identified, and the percentage of issues successfully addressed and completed. Initially, aggressive time frames to complete the priority issues were set, but have since been modified to better match the organization's priorities and resources. Overall themes arising in the

WalkArounds are also reviewed annually. Priority issues have tended to fall into two categories—(1) issues that have quick solutions, and (2) complex systemic and operational concerns that require significant analysis to better identify solutions that result in a sustainable improvement. Systemic and process failures require multiple levels of management to adequately resolve and are labeled as "require intervention" issues.

Integration and Spread

As Levtzion-Korach et al. noted, it is the combined knowledge from many reporting systems that builds optimal patient safety systems.[3] Using WalkArounds findings as one of numerous strategies to capture safety issues, cultural nuances, risk gaps, and learning is increasingly used within our organization. The overlap between safety reports, WalkArounds, surveys, complaints, and patient satisfaction reports guides the safety team to communicate findings, trends, and systemic gaps more effectively. This, in turn, informs management and empowers our decision makers to set clearer improvement goals.

In 2008 we hosted an Open House (in partnership with Ontario's Quality Healthcare Network[4]) for other local health care organizations to share our learning about WalkArounds and to contrast and compare our execution with models from other health care organizations. The interest and enthusiasm of the participating organizations demonstrated the timeliness of this program, and other health care organizations have in turn introduced their own experience-based adaptations.

Sustainability of WalkArounds

Sunnybrook Health Sciences Center made a further commitment to WalkArounds in 2007 by allocating a small facilities maintenance and equipment fund that can be accessed by the senior leaders to address small repairs or equipment requisitions that facilitate the resolution needs of the units. A risk-assessment code matrix was developed to uniformly assess need in a criteria-based manner.

In 2010 the University of Toronto's Centre for Patient Safety performed an evaluation of the WalkArounds process.[5] The evaluation findings directed the patient safety leaders to consider even better approaches to feedback and directing the conversations to root causes of local safety concerns. Changes to the process include (1) broader program-based representation, and (2) preselecting a topic to focus the discussion, which necessitates inviting subject matter experts to the WalkAround, who are able to contribute professional or support service content. The organization is currently piloting and evaluating these changes to the WalkArounds process.

The perception of WalkArounds as a useful tool will be sustained only by persistent attention to follow-up communication to the frontline staff participants and the spread of improvements to other units. As we uncover more complex system-level issues, we shall need to consider how best to leverage the benefits obtained on one unit to all units. The capability to annually reassess the WalkArounds process has allowed the coordinators to refine the roles of the stakeholders to remain alert to the changing needs and priorities of the organization.

References

1. Frankel A, et al. Patient Safety Leadership WalkRounds. *Jt Comm J Qual Saf.* 2003;29(1):16–26.
2. Vincent C, et al. How to investigate and analyse clinical incidents: Clinical risk unit and association of litigation and risk management protocol. *BMJ.* 2000 Mar 18;320(7237):777–781.
3. Levtzion-Korach O, et al. Integrating incident data from five reporting systems to assess patient safety: Making sense of the elephant. *Jt Comm J Qual Patient Saf.* 2010;36(9):402–410.
4. Quality Healthcare Network. Home page. Accessed Oct 21, 2012. http://www.qhn.ca/.
5. University of Toronto Centre for Patient Safety. Home page. Accessed Oct 31, 2012. http://www.patientsafetytoronto.ca.

to increase visibility or, at the discretion of the leaders or department, in a back room or empty patient room. There are advantages to each of these modes. If the discussion is held in the nursing station, staff working on the unit can observe the group in conversation and learn about the WalkRounds. The WalkRounds should be open for anyone to participate; hospitals that conduct the WalkRounds in an open area can stop clinicians who pass by and ask them to participate. If WalkRounds are conducted in a back room, such as a coffee lounge, participants are less likely to be pulled away for clinical issues. Interestingly, neither location seems detrimental to the candor of the conversation, and both modes are able to elicit comments on complex issues related to patient care and adverse events.

Sessions should include an opening statement (*see* Sidebar 5-4, page 50), and leaders should ask some detailed questions to prompt discussion. Questions may include the following:

- "What did we do that harmed a patient?"
- "How will we harm the next patient?"
- "What doesn't work well?"
- "What are you worried might happen that could hurt a patient?"
- "Do some ethnic groups get better care here than others?"
- "Do we disclose all that we reasonably should to patients, including mistakes and potential mistakes?"
- "How well does teamwork occur on this unit?"

These, and questions like these, will elicit different responses. For example, a night nurse might report that "At 5 A.M., an anticoagulated patient fell out of bed and hit her head and started bleeding. I paged four different physicians before I found the on-call physician. The patient lost a unit of blood." Other comments from employees may range from "The new bar-coding scanners won't accurately scan the IV bags again" to "The IV pole wheels were sticking. The patient tripped and cut her knee as a result. Her IV infiltrated at the same time."

The patient safety officer plays a critical role during the WalkRounds. He or she should ensure that only one conversation is conducted at any one time and help encourage quieter individuals to speak up. The senior leader can act as moderator if skilled and interested, but the patient safety officer should be responsible for, and capable of, making the rounds productive, inclusive, and focused.

Within the WalkRounds, all participants should be encouraged to give feedback. To ensure that all individuals are able to voice their concerns and that more reserved individuals will have an opportunity to speak, the patient safety officer or senior leader might consider asking the most junior individuals specifically about their concerns or take turns asking each individual in the group to comment on the topic being discussed.

During WalkRounds, the scribe should be taking notes. The scribe is one of, if not the most, critical participants in the WalkRounds process. It is his or her job to document information about what was said, who said it, and what the response was. Scribes in organizations performing WalkRounds have ranged from research assistants to the senior administrative assistant of the quality and safety department. Though a pad of paper will suffice for taking notes, many organizations use tabular forms that facilitate real-time sorting of concerns and start the process of distinguishing adverse events from their contributing factors. These forms should include the following fields:

- Date of WalkRound
- Location (unit, floor, and, if applicable, facility)
- Names of executives present
- Names of patient safety staff present
- For each comment, name of person speaking
- Concerns elicited from the unit on previous WalkRounds
- When elicited, contributing factors to concerns

Sidebar 5-4. Sample Opening and Closing Statements

Although opening and closing statements will vary among different organizations, following are sample statements used successfully across some organizations that conduct Executive WalkRounds.

Opening Statement

"We are moving as an organization to open communication and a just culture environment because we believe that doing so will make your work environment safer for you and your patients. The discussion we are interested in having with you is confidential and purely for patient safety and improvement. We are interested in focusing on the systems you work in each day rather than on blaming specific individuals. The questions we might ask you will tend to be general ones, and you might consider how these questions might apply in your work areas in regard to medication errors, communication or teamwork problems, distractions, inefficiencies, problems with protocols, and so forth. We are happy to discuss any issues of concern to you. Our goal is to take what we learn in these conversations and use them to improve your work environment and our overall delivery of care."

Closing Statement

"We appreciate the time and effort you put into taking care of patients and making their experience in our organization remarkable. Our job is to take the information you have given us, analyze it carefully, figure out what actions we might take to fix problems, assign those responsibilities to individuals, and hold their feet to the fire until the problems are solved. We promise to let you know how we're doing, and we will come back and elicit your opinion. We will work on the information you have given us. In return we would like you to tell two other people you work with about the concepts we have discussed in this conversation. As you see or think of other adverse events or are concerned about potential harm to a patient please report it by _____ (fill in the mechanism to be used in your organization). Near misses and adverse events are windows that we can all use to improve the safety of care we deliver. We can only address the issues if we know and talk about them openly."

Source: Allan Frankel. Used with permission.

- Status of any prior concerns

When the WalkRound has finished, the scribe will enter data collected into the database for further analysis.

After WalkRounds conclude, the executive team should immediately debrief on site (*see* information on debriefing in Chapter 6), assign urgent action items if needed, and together compare the scribe's notes with the

Sidebar 5-5. Using a Database to Track Information

Brigham and Women's Hospital in Boston has been using WalkRounds to identify patient safety issues for many years. To help sort, track, and analyze data collected during the WalkRounds, the team designed an Access database, which has been refined over a seven-year period and effectively used by other hospitals around the country. Demographic information can be entered into the database and correlated with events elicited during each WalkRound. Built into the database are templates for reports that can be structured in a manner useful for executive leadership or with greater detail for specific departments or managers.

The database tracks information from the time it is elicited during WalkRounds through the assignment of contributing factors, the identification of actions to be taken, notation for when action is taken, responsibility for follow-up, and final disposition. An action is deemed complete (problem resolved) or closed (addressed as fully as possible) only when it is communicated back to the front line and more specifically to the individual(s) who raised the issue during WalkRounds.

team's understanding of the issues. The scribe should add to his or her notes any other insights generated during this discussion. The group should discuss what went well, what went poorly, and what was learned, and possibly begin prioritizing important issues and potential improvements.

4. Tracking. To effectively track information gleaned during the WalkRounds process, organizations should set up a robust system for tracking and ranking collected data, such as an interactive database that allows for sorting and prioritizing (*see* Sidebar 5-5, above). Using a database, organizations can accomplish the following:

• Track names of individuals who participate in each WalkRound.

• Note location, time, and date of each round.

• Record comments given and hazards identified during the rounds.

• Identify the contributing factors.

• Develop actions to address the issues.

• Link specific comments with the individuals who initially discussed them.

• Link comments with those charged to fix them.

Within the tracking system, it may be beneficial to have a systemized way of ranking issues. This may involve

the previously mentioned severity/frequency approach (*see* page 43) or other method.

Information from the WalkRounds process should be integrated with other data, including reporting system, root cause analyses, surveillance, and audit data. The patient safety team is typically responsible for synthesizing data, integrating with other organizational data, and helping with prioritization. This involves categorizing WalkRounds comments, determining action items, presenting information to the multidisciplinary group, and tracking progress on any initiatives.

5. Reporting. After information has been entered and analyzed, organizations should share data with a multidisciplinary committee so that action items may be assigned to management personnel. Often the patient safety committee is the designated committee to receive WalkRounds information. Although this is often appropriate, the data collected from WalkRounds are frequently broader than "safety" alone and some link to an administrative and clinical operations group is required. From there, different committee members can take ownership of different projects or initiatives.

6. Feedback. A critical element to the WalkRounds process is a clearly delineated and formal structure for feedback to frontline providers who participate in WalkRounds, and to executive boards about findings and actions taken to address issues brought up in WalkRounds. By using formal methods of feedback, your organization can ensure the appropriate buy-in from all levels in the organization, foster commitment to the WalkRounds process, and facilitate planning, prioritization, and assignment of action items.

When communicating with the frontline staff, organizations should make it clear that staff members' comments are valued and will lead to change in care delivery. When you are just starting to implement WalkRounds, staff may be hesitant to report issues or may believe that the information reported is insubstantial or awkward. After the frontline providers and managers realize the benefits to be accrued— that improvements actually occur—the conversations become more open and robust. There are many effective ways to communicate with staff, including the following:

• Memos or e-mails to individual providers. Within such notes, you can thank staff for joining in the conversation, identify the major topics discussed, and review those slated for further analysis and action.

- Newsletter articles
- Periodic data summaries to managers for dissemination to staff
- Town hall meetings with executives to highlight accomplishments
- Dashboards that communicate the status of critical issues

Feedback should occur promptly. Even if action is delayed, the staff person should receive feedback on what is being done to address his or her issue. Organizations should deliver feedback in multiple and redundant ways to make sure the information is clearly visible, received, and understood by all.

Communication with executive boards can take the form of monthly reports to senior and physician leaders, quarterly reports to patient safety/quality committees, and biannual reports to boards.

7. Measurement. It is important to evaluate whether WalkRounds are effective in improving the organization's culture. As discussed in Chapter 2, a number of validated surveys are available to quantify caregivers' attitudes and perceptions of their working environments. WalkRounds have been directly linked with improvements in cultural perceptions and attitudes about teamwork, perceptions of management, willingness to speak up, and the overall safety of the working environment.[11,13]

REFERENCES

1. Bagian JP, et al. The Veterans Affairs root cause analysis system in action. *Jt Comm J Qual Improv.* 2002;28(10):531–545.
2. Frankel A, et al. Patient Safety Leadership WalkRounds. *Jt Comm J Qual Saf.* 2003;29(1):16–26.
3. Frankel A, et al. Patient Safety Leadership WalkRounds™ at Partners Healthcare: Learning from implementation. *Jt Comm J Qual Patient Saf.* 2005;31(8):423–437.
4. Hickson GB, et al. Balancing systems and individual accountability in a safety culture. In The Joint Commission: *From Front Office to Front Line: Essential Issues for Health Care Leaders,* 2nd ed. Oak Brook, IL: Joint Commission Resources, 2011, 1–35.
5. Chassin MR, Loeb JM. The ongoing quality improvement journey: Next stop, high reliability. *Health Aff (Millwood).* 2011;30(4):559–568.
6. Institute of Medicine. *To Err Is Human: Building a Better Health System.* Washington, DC: National Academy Press, 2000.
7. Marx D. *Patient Safety and the "Just Culture": A Primer for Health Care Executives.* New York City: Columbia University, 2001.
8. Marx D. How building a 'just culture' helps an organization learn from errors. *OR Manager.* 2003;19(5):1, 14–15, 20.
9. Nelson EC, et al. Microsystems in health care: Part 1. Learning from high-performing front-line clinical units. *Jt Comm J Qual Improv.* 2002;28(9):472–493.
10. Thomas EJ, et al. The effect of executive walk rounds on nurse safety climate attitudes: A randomized trial of clinical units. *BMC Health Serv Res.* 2005 Apr 11;5(1):28. Erratum in: *BMC Health Serv Res.* 2005 Jun 8;5(1):4.
11. Gandhi TK, et al. Closing the loop: Follow-up and feedback in a patient safety program. *Jt Comm J Qual Patient Saf.* 2005;31(11):614–621.
12. Shulkin DJ, Otten H. The walk-through patient-focus assessment: Preliminary results in augmenting patient satisfaction data. *Am J Med Qual.* 1993;8(2):68–71.
13. Frankel A, et al. Revealing and resolving patient safety defects: The impact of Leadership WalkRounds™ on frontline caregiver assessments of patient safety. *Health Serv Res.* 2008;43(6):2050–2066.

Chapter Six

EFFECTIVE TEAMWORK AND COMMUNICATION

Karen Frush, BSN, MD; Michael Leonard, MD; Allan Frankel, MD

Fundamentally, effective communication is the accurate exchange of information between two or more people. It can be formal or informal, brief or lengthy, detailed or vague. Failures in communication occur when the information exchange is not complete, effective, or appropriate. When such communication failures occur within the health care setting, the consequences can be severe. Treatments can be overlooked, diagnoses missed, risks not addressed, and patients hurt. In fact, the overwhelming majority of untoward events in medicine involve communication failures.

Common communication mishaps resulting in patient harm include the following:
- Providing care with incomplete or missing information
- Executing poor handoffs with relevant clinical data not clearly communicated
- Failing to confirm, or read back, information transmitted
- Failing to share and communicate known information, such as when a team member knows there is a problem, but is unable to speak up about it. For example, there are many documented cases of wrong-site surgery that show that someone in the room was aware the surgeon was operating on the incorrect site but was afraid to speak up about it.
- Assuming the expected outcome and safety of care. *Consider the following example: A patient arrives at a very good hospital for an elective total hip replacement. He is completely healthy and only takes one baby aspirin a day. Unexpectedly, a laboratory draw performed in the preoperative holding area shows the patient has severe thrombocytopenia, with 8,000 platelets/mL. Although this is a critical test result—it is much lower than the normal value of approx 150,000–200,000 platelets/mL—the laboratory fails to call in the result. Five skilled clinicians—the preoperative nurse (who is distracted with another patient), the surgical resident, the attending orthopedist, the nurse anesthetist, and the staff anesthesiologist—all miss the finding when they look through the chart. In fact, a spinal anesthetic is placed, which is completely contraindicated because of the risk of epidural hematoma. In the midst of surgery, with the patient in disseminated intravascular coagulation, someone in the lab notices the critical test result and calls the operating room. Things do not go well; for example, the surgeon is having great difficulty trying to stop the patient from bleeding.*

Creating an environment centered on effective communication offers several benefits, including the following:
- Contributes to the consistent delivery of high-quality, safe patient care
- Allows staff to learn from mistakes rather than placing individual blame—helping care providers understand how they work together effectively in a very complex environment
- Is essential in managing the complexity of patient care in a setting that often exceeds the capabilities of an individual clinician
- Ensures staff safety
- Enhances learning and opportunity for improvement
- Provides a more satisfying and rewarding work environment for staff
- Fosters an environment in which health care organizations can attract and retain critically important employees, such as nurses, pharmacists, and physicians
- Supports better interactions with patients and families, with higher patient satisfaction

WHY IS EFFECTIVE COMMUNICATION SO DIFFICULT IN HEALTH CARE?

Despite the importance of effective communication, ineffective communication is a pervasive problem in health care organizations. There are many possible reasons for this, including the following:

- Traditional health care culture has been characterized as one that values autonomy, hierarchy, and individual accomplishment and expertise. It should not be surprising then that many leaders have not prioritized effective communication and teamwork within their organizations. As discussed in Chapter 1, a high-performance culture based on structured and open communication cannot exist without visible and sustained leadership commitment. While it is easy for leaders to say "we must communicate better," to achieve such a culture leaders must be open and honest about errors, actively participate in initiatives to improve communication, incorporate effective communication into policies and procedures, specifically train professionals in better communication techniques, foster the creation and maintenance of teams, and hold everyone—including themselves—accountable for effective communication.

- Many health care professionals continue to place great value on autonomy and have trouble understanding the inherent value in teamwork.[1] As also discussed in Chapter 1, health care professionals have traditionally been trained to be individual experts who work hard to provide patient care.[2] The idea of working as a team, valuing multiple inputs, and solving problems collaboratively is not inherent in many providers' way of thinking. Similarly, many health care providers have not been trained to appreciate the value of effective leadership in creating an environment of mutual respect—an environment in which high-performing teams can thrive. How a leader "sets the stage" every time the team comes together is critically important to effective communication and teamwork.[3] A good leader is able to create an environment in which everyone knows the plan, feels valued, and has been invited to speak up and voice both suggestions and concerns. Systematically showing providers the value of working collaboratively needs to be an organizational goal. The philosophy of "if we all just come together and do our jobs" greatly increases the risk of an adverse event when working in a complex environment full of surprises.

- Certain hierarchies are present within health care that act as barriers to effective communication.[4] Anytime a physician interacts with a nurse, a pharmacist, or other physicians, hierarchy and power distances exist. The perceived degree of hierarchy has a profound effect on the willingness of people to speak up, particularly to question a decision or identify a problem. Being at the top of the clinical hierarchy, physicians are typically less aware of the issue and the interpersonal dynamics that are created. Good leaders actively work to flatten hierarchy, minimize power distances, and consistently engage all team members.[5,6]

- The current, fragmented health care model reinforces and tolerates unstructured and often poor communication. For communication to be effective, organizational processes and systems must support and set the expectation of effective communication. For example, processes that include a repeat-back to confirm information; include structured communication templates to ensure that all the information is present; and require all participants to be respected and encouraged to speak up foster effective communication. Conversely, processes that don't do this can actually reinforce poor communication and set up providers to fail.

- Failure of leadership to define and insist on an environment in which everyone is universally treated with respect. As noted in a Joint Commission *Sentinel Event Alert,* abusive and disrespectful behavior is dangerous. According to the *Alert,* "Intimidating and disruptive behaviors can foster medical errors, contribute to poor patient satisfaction and to preventable adverse outcomes, increase the cost of care, and cause qualified clinicians, administrators and managers to seek new positions in more professional environments."[7] If someone at the bedside is hesitant to voice concern about a patient or call someone because "it wasn't too much fun the last time we interacted," then there is an unacceptable risk. As previously mentioned, clearly defining that abusive and disrespectful behavior is out of bounds and enforcing such a policy is critical to creating a high-performance culture that delivers safe care.

Most health care providers have not been systematically taught how to effectively communicate, particularly across health care disciplines. Medical, nursing, pharmacy, and other health care–related schools focus on clinical information and scientific knowledge, but do not have a central focus on how to effectively communicate, interact, and respond to peers, patients, and other providers. This lack of standardized approach means the different disciplines enter the clinical care environment with different styles, their own jargon, and little knowledge about the inherent value in standardized and clear communication.

For example, nurses have historically been taught to be narrative in their communication—"tell a story." This has been reinforced by the traditional nursing edict—"you don't make diagnoses." Physicians, on the other hand, are systematically trained to give "the 10-second version, the headlines." It is not that any one style is right or wrong, but they are different, and having a common and predictable structure for communication is extremely important to help navigate those differences. To compensate for health care providers' lack of communication skills, certain strategies and tools can enhance communication and foster teamwork. Such strategies and tools can be effectively applied in all clinical health care domains, inpatient and outpatient. Following is a discussion of some of these strategies and tools.

Set the Tone for Teamwork

As previously mentioned, effective leaders set the stage for team interaction by creating and supporting an atmosphere in which people believe their input is valued and it is safe to ask questions, and they are comfortable speaking up if they don't understand or perceive a problem. Setting a positive tone for interaction can greatly promote cohesion and collaboration among individuals.[8,9] Conversely, a negative tone can inhibit communication and lead to error.

The team leader, consciously or unconsciously, sets the tone of collaboration very quickly—in about 5–10 seconds—through his or her verbal communication, body language, facial expressions, and attitude. It is critically important to set a tone that promotes psychological safety—where everyone on the team feels comfortable to speak up and voice concerns—and for the leader to share the plan so the team has clear goals. (*See* the following section for more information on psychological safety.)

Most health care team leaders are unaware of the importance of actively setting a positive tone and the behaviors associated with such activity. In an observational study of 300 surgical cases, researchers noticed that surgeons were critical to setting the tone for team interaction. As they prepared for the next surgical case, operating room (OR) team members—nurses, technicians, and anesthesia providers—participated in active dialogue about the case, social issues, and so forth before the surgeon entered the room. Within 10 seconds of entering the room, the surgeon's behavior had a profound effect on the communication pattern in the room. If the surgeon engaged the team, set a positive tone, and shared the plan, all the communication continued. However, if he or she set a negative tone, all team communication was virtually eliminated.[10]

Consider this example: An obstetrician known to be unpleasant to the nurses arrives to cover labor and delivery for the evening. She says, " I have a busy day tomorrow, so I really don't want to be called." Clearly the threshold to voice a concern or seek help has been seriously raised, producing an unsafe environment for the patients, the nurses, and the physician.

Most leaders set the stage for interactions informally or by default. A better idea is to actively set the stage with the message that "we're all contributing value to the care of this patient, this is a team sport, and we will work together in a respectful, open manner that encourages collaboration and welcomes input—and let's make this as enjoyable as we can." Team leaders can establish a positive tone immediately by greeting everyone by name and continuously inviting team members into conversation.

Ensure Psychological Safety

Within psychologically safe environments, everyone is comfortable speaking up, every individual and what they have to say is treated with respect at all times, and disrespectful actions are not tolerated.

Psychological safety is essential for teams[11]; people act tentatively and defensively when they don't feel safe, thereby inhibiting their willingness to participate and speak up. When team members believe that they or their suggestions are being criticized, a very unhealthy dynamic occurs, eroding team cohesion.

Nothing can erode psychological safety faster than a disrespectful colleague. Such disrespectful behavior can lead to a decrease in contributions from other colleagues, a decrease in task performance from other colleagues, and an increase in the general negative mood and anger of the room. In short, there is no place for unprofessional disruptive behavior in a team—it's dangerous.[12]

To ensure psychological safety, leaders must be explicit that overt disrespect is not acceptable and will not be tolerated. To do this, organizations must codify respect into the credentialing process and deal with violations to that code consistently and swiftly. Is leadership willing to codify this in the credentialing process and hold individuals equally accountable regardless of their standing and how much business they bring in? If so, a high-performance, safe culture can be achieved; if not, the chances of having a serious, avoidable, and potentially indefensible event rise dramatically.

Consider this example: An organization had been working with its entire clinical staff on teamwork and communication skills. The hospital had instituted multiple initiatives to improve communication, and organization leadership was proud of their accomplishments and believed that the organization supported teamwork and communication.

In the critical care unit, though all the staff had been educated regarding effective teamwork, the physicians and the nurses continued to hand off patients separately, and were quite resistant to finding ways to have effective multidisciplinary rounds. This lack of a forum to get the whole team "on the same page" generated many one-on-one conversations to clarify the plan of care for patients.

Compounding this problem was the fact that two of the intensivists often refused to respond to nurses' inquiries and would loudly and publicly proclaim "talk to the hand" or "come back and talk to me when you can ask a more intelligent question." This sent a destructive message that it was not psychologically safe to approach these physicians. No one wants to be treated disrespectfully or be humiliated in front of his or her peers. The attempts to improve teamwork and communication were seriously undermined by this behavior, which led to some adverse events because concerns were often not voiced.

If an organization believes in creating a safe work environment in which all employees are treated with respect at all times, then it needs to be very clear that management will consistently model those values, send the message that anything less is not acceptable, and actively intervene in a timely manner to deal with disrespectful behavior. Let's look at a different example:

An anesthesiologist came to a surgical floor to remove an epidural catheter being used for postoperative pain control. The nurse caring for the patient informed the anesthesiologist that the patient was unable to take pain medications by mouth and that the care team felt the patient would benefit from leaving the catheter in for another day or two. The anesthesiologist not only refused to acknowledge the nurse's multiple requests to leave the catheter intact, but pulled the catheter out while being rude to the nurse in front of the patient. Taking hospital leadership at its word that working collaboratively and treating each other *with respect was essential, six nurses called the CEO's office within 10 minutes of the incident. The CEO's response was immediate. The anesthesiologist was told in no uncertain terms to return to the floor and openly apologize to the nurse, and he did so within 30 minutes of the incident. This sent a very clear message that teamwork and communication were essential to the organization's culture.*

Use Structured Communication Techniques

Communication between individuals is often informal, disorganized, and variable. In situations where specific and complex information must be communicated and responded to in a timely manner, and the consequences of omitting critical information can be dire, it is essential to consistently add structure to the exchange. Such structure can ensure that the right information is shared at the right time with the right people. It also creates predictability as to how team members will communicate. Following are some specific structured communication techniques that all patient care teams should use:

Briefings

Briefings are a critical element in team effectiveness and determine whether people work together as a cohesive team or as a group of individuals with different ideas and goals sharing the same space. They quickly help set the tone for team interaction, ensure that people providing clinical care have a shared mental model of what's going to happen during a process, identify any risk points, plan for contingencies, and avoid surprises. When done effectively, briefings can establish predictability, reduce interruptions, prevent delays, and build social relationships and capital for future interactions.[13]

When structuring a briefing, it is important to keep in mind certain key elements, including the following (*see* Sidebar 6-1 on page 57 for a checklist for briefings):

• Be concise. For briefings to add value, they have to be seen as providing a positive return for the time spent. Meaningful information should be communicated quickly, enhancing operational efficiency, not hindering it.

• Involve others. Having a two-way conversation during a briefing is essential. Engaging others and explicitly asking for their input and suggestions brings more expertise to the issue at hand. A two-way conversation also offers an opportunity to assess people's comfort level and prior experience

---

Sidebar 6-1. Checklist for a Concise Briefing

Following is a checklist that team leaders can use to help ensure that a briefing is thorough yet concise:
✔ I got the other person's attention.
✔ I made eye contact and faced the person.
✔ I introduced myself and used people's names—familiarity is key.
✔ I shared the plan and asked for information they would know.
✔ I explicitly asked for input—both expertise and concerns.
✔ We talked about next steps.
✔ I encouraged ongoing monitoring and cross-checking.

Source: Leonard M, Graham S, Taggart B. The human factor: Effective teamwork and communication in patient strategy. In Leonard M, Frankel A, Simmonds T, editors: *Achieving Safe and Reliable Healthcare: Strategies and Solutions.* Chicago: Health Administration Press, 2004, 37–64.

---

relative to a clinical task. Having team members participate enhances team formation and clarifies that everyone has a responsibility to ensure safe care and speak up if they perceive something to be unsafe. Effective leaders always think out loud to share the plan, and by continually inviting team members into the conversation for their ideas and concerns, they make themselves approachable.[14]

• Use first names. Familiarity is a key factor in the willingness of people to speak up when they perceive a problem. Using people's names is also a sign of respect. If you are in an environment in which people don't know each other, write names on a whiteboard for reference.

• Make eye contact and face the person. As the Buddhists would say—be in the moment. Acknowledging others and paying attention to what they say sends a positive message, thus reinforcing that their contributions have value and importance. It is important to note that eye contact should be exercised when working with individuals who are culturally comfortable with it. Some cultures view direct eye contact as a threat, and thus it should be avoided in situations where a team member is uncomfortable.[15]

Although briefings can and should be done in almost any situation, there are some environments in which briefings are particularly important, including the following:

• In procedural areas. In this environment, briefing prior to each procedure should be done. As previously mentioned, such briefing should include a discussion of the plan, contingencies to the plan, possible risk points, and so forth. As

part of its Universal Protocol for Preventing Wrong Site, Wrong Procedure, Wrong Person Surgery™, The Joint Commission requires surgical teams to conduct a specific type of preprocedure briefing—typically called a time-out—in which the correct site, patient, and procedure are verified. This briefing is also an opportunity to address other issues such as antibiotic administration, medications, allergies, access to critical equipment, anticipated problems, and other salient issues.

The World Health Organization (WHO) Surgical Safety Checklist for preprocedure briefings helps the surgical team coordinate discussions about safety during various phases of the surgical continuum.[16] Yet another preprocedure briefing tool is the High-5 Correct Site Surgery Standard Operating Protocol,[17] which requires certain preoperative checks, surgical site marking, and a "time out" before surgery.

The Universal Protocol, WHO Surgical Safety Checklist, and High-5 Correct Site Surgery Standard Operating Protocol are all intended to improve the safety of surgical procedures. As a result, they have many features in common. While they are not identical, they are compatible with each other. The Universal Protocol and the High-5 Protocol focus specifically on reducing the risk of wrong-patient, wrong-procedure, and wrong-site surgery. The High-5 Protocol applies to certain types of surgical cases and requires participating hospitals to adhere to the protocol as written, to measure their performance and share their results. In contrast, the WHO Surgical Safety Checklist addresses a much broader array of surgical risks, is available to any organization wishing to use it, and is presented as a model tool that may be modified at the user's discretion to fit local practice. Evidence suggests that use of the WHO Surgical Safety Checklist is associated with significant reductions in postoperative complication rates and death rates.[18,19]

Where the three methodologies overlap—certain preoperative checks, site marking, and the "time-out" before surgery—the expectations are consistent. Where they differ is in the range of perioperative activities included in each. The High-5 Protocol has a more fully developed preoperative verification process that begins when the surgical procedure is first scheduled and continues throughout the preoperative process, while the WHO Surgical Safety Checklist and the Universal Protocol are initiated preoperatively on the day of surgery. On the other hand, the WHO

Surgical Safety Checklist includes a postoperative "sign out" process that is not part of the High-5 Protocol. All of these components have value and, indeed, should be implemented by all organizations providing surgical services.

The Dutch SURPASS (Surgical Patient Safety System), a patient-specific multidisciplinary checklist that covers the entire surgical-patient pathway, is used to assess whether surgical patients receive consistent care from the time they are scheduled for surgery throughout the hospital stay and onto discharge. The results of this program are nothing short of remarkable. Surgical mortality in the six intervention hospitals decreased from 1.5% to 0.8% (47%) and complications, decreased from 27.3% to 16.7% (39%). The number of patients requiring a second surgical procedure to resolve a complication or suffering a temporary disability also decreased. Outcomes did not change in the five control hospitals.[20]

Having a systematic process creates predictability and helps ensure that patients receive consistent care. It is important to note that SURPASS is not "cookbook medicine," in which clinicians are told how to provide care. What it does provide is a predictable process by default, which still allows for skilled clinicians to deviate and change care if they feel that is indicated. Acknowledging clinical expertise is critical for cultural acceptance, and the overall process allows for measurable improvement.

SURPASS has been implemented in 40 hospitals in the Netherlands, with the intent to spread it to every hospital in the country. Its use has enabled the identification of more than 6,000 defects—roughly 1,000 in surgery, 2,000 preoperatively, and 3,000 postoperatively.[21]

In addition to a preprocedure briefing, team members should consider spending a few minutes at the beginning of the day to look across the schedule, anticipate equipment and supply needs, and plan for contingencies. This is not only time well spent, but it allows each preprocedural briefing to be shorter, can prevent delays in starting procedures, and can minimize interruptions during procedures. There are times when procedures are significantly delayed because the team doesn't have all the tools, equipment, and supplies it needs for the operation. Sometimes a specific tool is not even in the hospital, and the procedure is held up while the tool is brought on site. This can be a risk to patient safety and is completely preventable. By conducting a briefing before the start of a schedule, team members can identify

what special equipment and supplies are needed, and that equipment and those supplies can be brought in before the procedure begins. (*See* Sidebar 6-2, above.) Such planning can also minimize the need for the circulating nurse to leave the OR to retrieve necessary equipment and supplies during a procedure. When a circulating nurse leaves the OR, it is not only a distraction to the procedure but may present an infection control risk as well.[22]

• In the ICU. Given the intensity and frequently changing nature of the patient needs in the ICU, it is important that teams come together at the beginning of the day and periodically throughout the day to talk about patients, plans of care, possible risk points, and issues to watch. This can help all team members get on the same page and see the big picture of which patients need what care in what time frame. The use of multidisciplinary rounds and setting daily goals for each patient should be a fundamental goal in the ICU.[23] (*See* page 64 for more information on multidisciplinary rounds.)

• In ambulatory care. With the high volume and short intervals involved with this type of care, it is constructive to take a few minutes in the morning to brief the day's activities. Within such a briefing, some things to discuss could include here's who's coming in, here's who we're concerned about, and here's the information we need. Team members should identify which patients' care should be simple, and who is probably going to be complicated. They can also talk about what their resources are regarding personnel, competing tasks, and any anticipated personnel shortages. In addition to the morning briefing, the team should briefly reconnect at points throughout the day to address questions such as How are we doing on time? Who's new? What's different? What's changed? This helps keep everyone in "the same movie," a set of shared context and expectations. Such a briefing is much more effective than the typical one-on-one hallway conversations that can occur within the ambulatory care setting.

• On the spot/as the situation changes. If something significantly changes in the course of patient care, team leaders should take a few moments to make sure everyone is working off a common mental model. Every team member should feel comfortable with gathering the team together for one or two minutes if the "game changes." Some high-performing units actually set the expectation that team members are required to speak up under these circumstances.

• Handoffs. These occur when patient care is transferred from one team member to another. These are inherently dangerous times, as critical information can be lost, forgotten, or misinterpreted during handoffs. Handoffs may take place in a variety of situations. They may involve one service taking over for another in the emergency department, such as gynecology for general surgery with a patient with pelvic pain; or a physical handoff, such as moving from the post-operative recovery room to the ICU. A very important handoff is the patient moving from a primary care environment into the hospital and back. Effective handoffs in this circumstance can lessen avoidable complications and unexpected hospital readmissions. No matter the type of handoff, it is important that pertinent information is effectively communicated and does not get lost in the shuffle. Unfortunately, this doesn't always happen.

The transition of patient care through the handoff process is prone to communication error and inadequate clinical content. Communication errors can lead to sentinel events as can be seen in data from The Joint Commission, which identifies communication as the third leading root cause in sentinel events reported between 2004 and 2011.[24] To address the issue of poor communication in care transitions, The Joint Commission requires a standardized approach to handoff communications: Element of Performance (EP) 2, "The hospital's process for hand-off

communications provides for the opportunity for discussion between the giver and receiver of patient information," in Provision of Care (PC) Standard PC.02.02.01 ("The hospital coordinates the patient's care, treatment, and services based on the patient's needs").[25]

Similarly, in 2011 the Accreditation Council on Graduate Medical Education (ACGME) revised its Common Program Requirements regarding communication during care transitions after it began receiving increased reports of ineffective communication and cross-coverage problems. The number of handovers increased among residents when duty-hour restrictions were implemented in 2003.[26] In addition to requiring that clinical assignments minimize the number of transitions in patient care, the ACGME further requires that (1) GME programs ensure and monitor effective, structured handover processes to facilitate both continuity of care and patient safety; and (2) programs ensure that residents are competent in communicating with team members in the handoff process.[27]

In response to these types of requirements, some institutions have initiated standard education on and evaluation (observation) of the handoff process.

When designing a handoff process, keep in mind that the use of structured language can help ensure effective communication (*see* pages 60–61). In addition, tools such as checklists can be used to make sure all the appropriate information is communicated every time.

Debriefings

While briefings typically occur before a process, procedure, schedule of procedures, and so forth, a debriefing is a concise exchange that occurs after such events have been completed to identify what happened, what was learned, and what can be done better next time.[13] It is a valuable opportunity (rarely used in medicine) to determine how participants in a team are feeling about the process and to identify opportunities for improvement, as well as to further education and learning. Debriefing is also an effective venue for problem solving and generating new solutions—often with ideas brought from other clinical domains by the experts on the team. It is a very good way to positively engage the collective wisdom of a care team. Finally, as recently demonstrated, debriefing—as well as briefing—can be used to prospectively surface clinical and operational defects in surgical care, and thereby prevent patient harm. In a 44-month-period, surgical teams, using a one-page, double-sided briefing and debriefing tool, identified a total of 6,202 defects—an average of 141 defects per month; equipment (48%) and communication (31%) issues were most prominent.[28]

For the debriefing process to work well, there needs to be psychological safety. If staff members don't feel safe to speak up, they won't. It is essential that the debriefing conversation is all about opportunity and learning. Blame and judgment will kill the debriefing process very quickly. Note that any concerns with a team member's behavior or performance should be an individual conversation, never a public one.

The effectiveness of a debriefing is dependent on the effectiveness of the briefing. If you weren't clear at the front end, you won't be able to effectively wrap up the information. The debriefing conversation should be focused on the common goal and have a positive tone. In facilitating a debriefing, team leaders should be as specific as possible. It's nice to say "nice job," but not much is learned. The more specific and detailed, the more value will be gained. Appropriate questions to ask during debriefing include the following:

• What did we do well? Focus on both individual and team tasks.

• What did we learn?

• What would we do differently next time?

• Were there system issues, such as equipment problems or incomplete information, that made our job more difficult? Who's going to own the system problems so they will get fixed and not be a recurrent pebble in our shoe?

During debriefing it is important to engage the most junior team members first. If you engage the 20-year veteran nurse first, and she says she did not see any issues, the nurse fresh out of nursing school will likely be hesitant to bring up an issue. However, if you ask the recent graduate first, you not only encourage him or her to speak freely and identify potential issues, but you also help him or her learn and grow professionally.

After a debriefing, teams should document items that did not go well and make suggestions for improvement. By capturing and documenting problems, teams can take a step toward fixing them and preventing issues down the line. (*See* Chapter 13 for a description of a learning system that can serve as a mechanism to track and act on information captured in the debriefing.)

In addition to identifying problems to fix, debriefings can speed up team learning. Such learning can occur regardless of the experience of the team leader. For example, a study by Edmondson, Bohmer, and Pisano showed that, when learning a new cardiac surgery procedure, the team that had the shortest learning curve and the best outcomes was led by a junior cardiac surgeon. This was due in part to the surgeon's conducting a debriefing after every operation and his creation of an environment of organizational learning within his team. The teams that did not engage in debriefing and collaborative learning had suboptimal outcomes.[8]

SBAR Model

An acronym for Situation, Background, Assessment, Recommendation, this structured communication technique is used to standardize communication between two or more people,[29] thereby promoting a focus on teamwork rather than individual expertise. It helps set the expectation within a conversation that specific, relevant, and critical informational elements are going to be communicated every time a patient is discussed. The SBAR model is particularly helpful in situations in which a nurse-physician encounter must occur. It helps get both parties on the same page, as the physicians want to focus on the problem and the solution, and the nurses know they will be expected to relate specific aspects of the problem. SBAR sets the expectation that critical thinking associated with defining the patient's problem and formulating a solution occur before the physician is contacted. Thus both parties know that the conversation will include the assessment and recommendation for care that is relevant to the patient's current status.

Following is a description of steps involved in SBAR:

• *Situation.* This is the part of the mechanism in which the two parties communicating establish the topic of which they are going to speak.

• *Background.* This is any information needed to make an informed decision for the patient, including the following:

—The admitting diagnosis and date of admission

—List of current medications, allergies, intravenous fluids, and labs

—Most recent vital signs

—Lab results, with the date and time the test was performed, and results of previous tests for comparison

—Other clinical information

—Code status

• *Assessment.* The individual initiating the SBAR should state an assessment of the situation and the patient's status.

• *Recommendation.* The individual initiating the SBAR should offer a recommendation of what to do next and when it should happen.

The following dialogue illustrates how a respiratory therapist can use the SBAR model to communicate with a physician regarding a patient's situation:

> • *Situation.* "I'm calling about Ms. Jones, who is short of breath."
> • *Background.* "She's a patient with chronic lung disease; she's been sliding downhill; and she's now acutely worse."
> • *Assessment.* "She has decreased breath sounds on the right side. I think she's probably collapsed a lung."
> • *Recommendation.* "I think she needs a chest tube. I need you to come see her now. When will you be here? What would you like me to do until you get here? What can I do to get ready?"

In this example, the respiratory therapist effectively communicates using the SBAR model. The communication is concise, clear, and resulted in timely action.

Assertive Language

Because medicine has an inherent hierarchical structure and power distances between individuals, it is critically important that health care workers politely assert themselves in the name of safety. Effective assertion is pleasant and persistent; it is not a license to be aggressive, hostile, or confrontational. This type of communication is also timely, clear, and offers solutions to presenting problems.

As previously mentioned, numerous high-profile accidents in medicine and elsewhere have demonstrated that in many cases team members knew that "something didn't seem right," but their ability to speak up and clearly communicate was inhibited. Often, the information was relayed in an oblique and indirect manner. The whole concept of "hint and hope"—"I said something, they must have heard it, and everything will be OK"— is all too common.

When assertion is ineffective, a look back usually reveals the following:

• Concern was expressed.

• The problem was stated in an oblique and indirect way.

• A proposed action didn't happen.

• A decision was not reached.

Organizations can help ensure appropriate assertion in team communication by training staff in assertion techniques. A formal checklist can be used to help staff learn a positive way to assert their opinions. Following is an example of such a checklist:

• Get the person's attention.

• Make eye contact, face the person.

• Use the person's name.

• Express concern.

• State the problem clearly and concisely.

• Propose action.

• Make sure the problem and proposed action are understood by all parties.

• Reassert as necessary.

• Reach a decision.

• Make sure the decision is understood by all parties—do a read-back.

• Escalate if necessary.

By following this checklist, staff members can ensure that their point is made. An individual may not always get the decision he or she wants, but at least everyone will be having the same conversation. It may be helpful to practice using this type of checklist during role-playing exercises.

Critical Language

During a stressful situation, such as a surgical procedure or an intense patient care episode, not everyone will immediately be able to think of the most appropriate way to get someone's attention and communicate information effectively—particularly if the person who needs to say something is hesitant to speak up due to hierarchy issues, his or her cultural background, or a lack of psychological safety.

Often providers, such as physicians, may not be aware of a situation, and nondirect language may not be strong enough to signal a problem. For this reason, it can be helpful to empower professionals with critical language that when spoken indicates to other team members that work should cease and all attention should be focused on the speaker. Such language may include a phrase like "I need a little clarity," a wonderful, neutral term that came from Allina Hospitals. A request for "clarity" can be used in the presence of a patient and his or her family, and all caregivers know that what is really being said is "let's just take a minute and make sure we are doing the right thing." Teams that respond to critical language know there is a concern that needs to be immediately addressed, and all work should cease until that situation is resolved.

Critical language should be neutral, help focus on doing the right thing, and foster a situation in which no one believes that their competence or expertise is being questioned.

Consider this example: A child comes into a pediatric clinic with an exacerbation of asthma. The medical assistant who brings the patient to the examination room is quite concerned that the child is struggling to breathe. As the medical assistant leaves the exam room, the pediatrician is walking down the hall to see another patient. The medical assistant says, "I have a child with asthma in room 2," but the busy physician doesn't stop to ask how serious the asthma is and walks off. The medical assistant waits a few minutes, becomes progressively more uncomfortable, and walks to the other end of the clinic to get a nurse. The nurse takes one look at the patient and interrupts the physician to come immediately. The child is taken emergently to the hospital. Use of critical language would have immediately captured the busy physician's attention and quite possibly prevented a delay in caring for the child.

Common Language

In some settings, using a common language, which is agreed upon by all providers in that setting, to describe critical issues or observations may be helpful to ensure consistency yet comprehensiveness in communication. For example, within the obstetrics setting, communication about fetal heart tracing can often be confusing and misleading. Different providers have different ways of expressing concern. When a fetal tracing indicates a problem, providers must move quickly and efficiently. Wasting time deciphering what someone means is not a luxury that the situation affords. To help clarify communication among providers about fetal heart tracings, the National Institute of Child Health and Human Development has defined an agreed-upon common language in obstetrics that describes such tracings.[30] When all providers use this language to objectively describe what they observe, organizations can ensure consistent communication about a critical issue within many different types of situations.

Closed Communication Loops

A closed communication loop, or read-back, helps improve the reliability of communication by having the person receiving the communication restate what the sender has said to confirm understanding. One specific type of closed-loop communication is repeat-back. The tool involves four distinct actions:

1. The "sender" concisely states information to the "receiver."

2. The receiver then repeats back what he or she heard.

3. The sender then acknowledges that the repeat-back was correct or makes a correction.

4. The process continues until a shared understanding is verified. Within this model, responding to a message with an "okay" or an "uh-huh" is not sufficient to close the communication loop. The message must be explicitly restated and acknowledged. We do this all the time in our personal lives when we order a latte or Chinese food over the phone. There is no reason we should not do it when patients are entrusting their well-being to us.

Organizations that mandate this type of closed-loop communication during times in which communication must be reliable and effective can help smooth the communication process and ensure that no critical information is lost. Closed-loop communication can be particularly helpful during surgery to confirm sponge count, during high-risk patient handoffs to ensure comprehensive information exchange, and during medication ordering to ensure that the right medication, right dose, and right route are communicated. The Joint Commission, for example, requires organizations to use a read-back closed-communication process when confirming verbal or telephone orders. One such requirement is EP 20 of Standard PC.02.01.03, which states, "Before taking action on a verbal order or verbal report of a critical test result, staff uses a record and 'read back' process to verify the information."[25]

Active Listening

A critical component of communication is listening. If providers do not listen to one another, then they can't effectively exchange information. Conversation is a two-way exercise involving both speaking and listening. Active listening is a concept in which a provider approaches the act of listening in the following way:

• Maintains a comfortable level of eye contact

• Monitors body language—both his or her own and the speaker's—to ensure that the correct messages are being sent and received

- Listens completely without framing a response while the individual is still speaking
- Repeats back information to confirm understanding

Callouts

Typically used in procedural settings, callouts involve clearly spoken phrases that indicate a phase of a process. This technique is often used in the OR at two points—the start of a procedure and the closing. Surgical teams may also use the callout technique at other times, such as to say the sponge count is correct or the patient is coming off bypass. Further examples of callouts include the following:

- "The waiting room is full of flu patients, we're getting behind."
- "X-ray is getting backed up, the wait for a CT scan is now 60 minutes."
- "We'll be done with this procedure in 30 minutes."
- "We're bleeding more than I like—we may need to open this patient. We'll decide within five minutes."

When using the callout technique, participants should speak clearly and loudly so all team members can hear.

Create Situational Awareness

Situational awareness (SA) is defined as a shared understanding of "what's going on," "what is likely to happen next," and "what to do if what is supposed to happen doesn't."[5] SA requires that team members have a common mental model of what is really expected. By maintaining SA, the care team creates a common understanding of what they are trying to accomplish; monitors and reports progress or potential problems; and avoids "tunnel vision"—becoming fixated on a particular task rather than the "larger picture"—to ensure that progress conforms to the shared model.

Within a complicated and hectic health care process, such as a surgical procedure or an ICU intervention, SA is easily lost, and the risk of accidents and problems goes up dramatically. Certain "red flags" can indicate the loss or potential loss of SA, and the presence of any of the following red flags should alert team members that risk is increasing and should be discussed.[5]

- Things don't feel right. This is probably the most important indicator of a problem. Expert individuals "pattern-match" against previous experience.[31] If intuition is telling an individual there is a problem, then the chances are quite good that the team is getting into trouble. If the hair on the back of his or her neck is standing up, or he or she is getting a bad feeling about what's going on, then the individual should verbalize any concerns to other team members so the problem can be addressed.
- Ambiguity. If it is becoming less clear what the plan is, then the team needs to talk to make sure everyone is on the same page. It's hard to monitor the plan if team members are not sure what is supposed to be happening.
- Reduced/poor communication. Faced with a problem, effective teams and leaders consciously enhance and increase communication. Raising concerns, gathering input, agreeing on how to approach problems, and having team members verify results should increase during problematic situations. A simple marker of this is active communication: "thinking out loud."
- Confusion
- Trying something new under pressure. This reflects the sense that the practitioner(s) does not have a workable approach to the problem at hand. Teams are far more successful staying with the tried-and-true approach, used many times before, than launching into novel approaches under duress. This is not to say being creative and innovative is not a positive attribute; however, when a team is behind the curve, they should do what they do best.
- Deviating from established norms. Norms have been established because they often reflect safe approaches to care. Unless there is a clear and compelling benefit discussed and clarified by the team, this can be an indicator of a problem.
- Verbal violence. This is a proxy for frustration. Effective communication becomes difficult when someone is being verbally unpleasant. It also affects people's comfort level in speaking up or questioning the current approach.
- Fixation. When people become task fixated, they lose the ability to see the context of the situation. An example of this would be the physician who is so fixated on getting the difficult central line in that he fails to notice the patient is becoming hypoxic or unstable.
- Boredom. It takes conscious work to maintain vigilance and attention. When one is bored, it is easy for the mind to wander from the task at hand. Being on autopilot is a good way to miss critical information.
- Task saturation. Being busy and feeling overwhelmed indicates a need to ask for help and communicate with other team members. Being behind the curve and working hard to

keep up narrows an individual's ability to process important information.

• Being rushed/behind schedule. In today's busy world of medical practice, everyone feels rushed or behind at some point. The danger with this situation is that it is human nature to cut corners when behind, and something important may be missed. Given that being rushed is encountered frequently, the safest answer is for individuals to check in with fellow team members to see that they are not missing something that could adversely affect patient care.

Building and maintaining SA is a collective process involving the entire team. Teams that take the following actions can establish and maintain SA:

• Communicate in a concise, specific, and timely manner.

• Use briefings, ongoing updates, and rebriefings to ensure that every team member knows the game plan.

• Acknowledge and demonstrate common understanding using repeat-back procedures.

• Talk to one another as events unfold so the team can monitor and verify perspectives.

• Anticipate the next steps and discuss possible contingencies.

• Constructively assert opinions and perspectives.

• Verbalize red flags if they are present.

STRUCTURES THAT ENHANCE TEAMWORK AND COMMUNICATION

In addition to the previously mentioned strategies and skills, organizations can and should establish structures in which effective teamwork and communication can take place. Following is a discussion of three such structures.

Multidisciplinary Rounds

An effective way to incorporate all the previously mentioned structured communication techniques is to use multidisciplinary rounds. These are rounds in which every member of the care team is present and every patient is discussed. When possible, the patient and family are included on these rounds. In the hospital, the bedside is the optimal location for these rounds. Such rounds should take place at least twice a day at shift changes, and an abbreviated version should occur throughout the day to address new developments, changes, or problematic situations. Within these

rounds, teams should discuss the plan of care for each patient.

In a busy clinic, getting the team together for multidisciplinary rounds, or a briefing, can be quite helpful to frame the day and get everyone in the same mental model. Multidisciplinary rounding allows the team to be proactive and think ahead, rather than reacting to events and experiencing surprises.

As previously mentioned, teams can use structured communication techniques, such as SBAR, briefings, and common language, to facilitate and streamline rounding conversations. Teams may also consider using whiteboards to spur discussion of every patient.

Although rounding can be effective in many different environments, it can be particularly useful in the obstetrics department and emergency department. Within these two departments, staff cannot control patient volume or workload and thus can benefit from periodically coming together, discussing risks, anticipating problems, and communicating when the workload is getting to be too much. When a staff member is feeling overwhelmed by his or her patient load, he or she should feel empowered to speak up during rounds, so work can be reallocated to ensure the safety of patients.

Nonnegotiable Agreed-on Norms of Conduct

In high-risk environments, there are a few situations in which the "right thing" is done every time. In our personal lives, most states have mandated seat belt use, as survival drops dramatically when humans become projectiles. In the Kaiser Permanente work in perinatal safety, it is agreed that "if the nurse or midwife asks a physician to come see a patient, the physician comes, 100% of the time, and with a good attitude."[32] In surgery, two important agreed-on norms are that anytime the sponge or instrument count is off, an x-ray will be taken, and the surgical team will not operate on a patient without verifying that they are doing the correct procedure on the correct patient at the correct site.

It is essential to have a short list of things that happen 100% of the time and have clear and logical consequences if they are not done. There's no such thing as partial credit in these areas. Note that having too many is not wise as they could be seen as "top down" mandates and less likely to be followed.

Mechanisms for Conflict Resolution

Health care teams always need to act in the best interest of the patient, but often they are not effective in resolving differences of opinion in an appropriate and respectful manner. In a culture in which people keep score by knowing the answer and being right, a consistent mechanism to anchor the conversation toward the common goal is important. This is a basic tenet of effective negotiation. The common goal in medicine is providing optimal, safe care for every patient, every time. By focusing on that goal and framing the conversation around that goal, we reiterate the goal, and move the team conversation to the "third person"—going from "who's right" and "who's wrong" or "who's in charge" to "here's what's right for the patient."[33] Conversations focused on who's right and who's wrong often do not end well, and increase the risk for the patient. Healthy cultures have effective mechanisms for resolving conflict so that all members of the team feel that they were heard and what is the best for the patient is the end result every time, as illustrated in the following example:

After talking with a patient, a nurse in the radiology suite was concerned that the informed consent form signed by the physician was incorrect. The patient was expecting a biopsy of the left lung, and the informed consent described a biopsy of the right lung. The nurse raised the concern to the physician, who responded that he was sure that the informed consent was correct. When the nurse respectfully but firmly restated her concern on behalf of the patient, the physician reviewed the patient's record and spoke with the patient. The physician then realized that an error had indeed been made, and the consent form was revised to describe the correct-side biopsy.

Comprehensive Unit-Based Safety Program (CUSP)

Establishing a multidisciplinary safety team is another way to promote effective teamwork and communication among health care providers. The Comprehensive Unit-Based Safety Program (CUSP) provides a model for structuring such a team, and this program has been adopted in many institutions.[23] CUSP was designed to improve safety culture and help providers learn from mistakes by integrating safety practices into the daily work of a clinical unit or care area. Foundational to this program is the creation of a multidisciplinary team, consisting of a nurse leader, a physician champion, representatives of other health care professionals who work on the unit (for example, a pharmacist, a respiratory therapist), and others involved in the work of the unit (unit clerk, technician, infection control expert, and so on). This team meets regularly to identify and solve "local" safety concerns, while at the same time aligning its work with safety and quality improvement goals set by institutional leaders.

The CUSP model is composed of five steps, which are designed to support continuous improvement by integrating evidence-based practices at the unit level:

Step 1: Educate the team and staff on the science of safety—This education includes such topics as safety as a property of the system; principles of safe design; and principles of high performing teams.

Step 2: Identify safety concerns (finding defects)—Safety concerns, risks, and defects can be identified through safety reporting systems, from sentinel event and harm data, and from "local knowledge" about risks to patients in that unit.

Step 3: Conduct WalkRounds with hospital executive leadership—As discussed in Chapter 5, WalkRounds are designed to open lines of communication between frontline providers and leaders, educate leaders about clinical issues and safety risks, provide staff with resources to mitigate risk, and hold staff accountable for improving patient safety.

Step 4: Implement improvements (learning from defects)—The CUSP model has a "learning from defects" tool, which is designed to help staff answer the following questions about the identified defect: (1) What happened? (2) Why did it happen? (3) What was done to reduce risk? (4) How do you know risks were actually reduced? The team is encouraged to learn from at least one defect per month.

Step 5: Document and share (spread) results—The unit-based safety team is asked to document, track, and audit identified safety concerns and provide updates at their monthly meetings. Progress can be reported to staff through bulletin boards, newsletters, staff meetings, and huddles. Results are also reported to hospital leaders through patient safety and quality committees, or directly at senior staff meetings by executives involved in WalkRounds.

The Joint Commission expects accredited hospitals to conduct an annual measure of safety culture,[25] and this type of baseline measurement should be obtained before implementing CUSP. Each clinical unit should then use its own culture data to monitor changes in patient safety and teamwork scores as CUSP is initiated and implemented. It is important to remember that culture change takes time, and improvements in safety and teamwork climate scores may not be seen for 12–18 months after CUSP is implemented.

TRAINING FOR EFFECTIVE TEAMWORK AND COMMUNICATION

Strong team performance with an emphasis on two-way communication, respect, idea sharing, and problem solving is essential to the safe and reliable delivery of care. Not only do health care teams not typically have this type of interaction, but many members of the team are unaware of how poor their communication and team behaviors are. For example, if you ask a physician if communication in care teams is effective, he or she will mostly likely say "yes." However, if you ask nurses the same question, you will get a different answer. In fact, 25%–40% of nurses surveyed in a cultural assessment tool said that they would be hesitant to speak up if they saw a physician making a mistake.[34] Part of the reason for this is that physicians and nurses view teamwork differently. Nurses believe that teamwork reflects the opportunity to provide input and feedback. Whereas physicians in high-performing units define teamwork as collaborative work based on respect and common goals. Some physicians in low-performing units state that teamwork means that everyone does what they say—not a functional or sustainable model.[34]

Effective teamwork and communication skills are not necessarily something a person is born with. Yes, there are those truly gifted individuals who have almost a sixth sense about what to say when and how. However, for the rest of us, communication strategies and teamwork skills can and should be taught, practiced, and reinforced until they become second nature and a critical part of how we operate. Unfortunately, in medicine, teamwork and communication skills have not commonly been included in the curriculum of medical, nursing, pharmacy, or other health care schools. And so the responsibility for such education falls on the health care organization.

Although research has shown a link between effective teamwork and improved patient outcomes, the evidence is less clear regarding what forms of training are most effective.[35] Questions remain as to what content to teach, what teaching methods have the most benefit, and how training should be evaluated. Overall, there is still much to learn regarding how to implement a feasible training program that leads to measurable changes in clinicians' teamwork behaviors.[36]

It is tempting to simply initiate team training in a clinical area without thoroughly assessing the environmental context. To achieve lasting improvement, however, several key success factors should be considered. First, it is critical that leadership in clinical units be supportive of teamwork training. If leaders do not value and reinforce the principles being taught, success is unlikely. Second, teamwork training seems to have a greater likelihood of success when there are local (for example, on the unit) champions of the effort who will support and reinforce the lessons learned. And last, team training has the most positive impact when participants use principles of effective communication to make positive process changes to support teamwork locally. Examples may include using whiteboards to share team member names or clarifying policies regarding key data that must be communicated in handoffs.

When training providers on teamwork and communication, consider bringing them together in multidisciplinary sessions to communicate the need for teamwork and communication; educate them on team behaviors, communication strategies, and structures for communication using scenarios they understand and can relate to; and have them practice using the behaviors and strategies. With this approach, two things happen. One is procedural learning—"I have done this, and I know how to do it well." This is extremely important in a culture that keeps score by knowing the answers and doing things well. People are far more likely to do something back at the bedside if they have practiced.

The second thing that happens is social agreement. When physicians, nurses, and technicians discuss a real case and how they would communicate about it and respond, they reach consensus about the appropriate communication pattern and practice together. When they use these teamwork behaviors where they deliver care, the fact that "we did this together before and agreed how we're going to do it" is very important to consistently embed team behaviors. This is very powerful in forming and enhancing relationships, the foundation of a safer culture.

As discussed in Chapter 2, before officially starting a training session, you may want to consider administering the safety culture survey. Realizing a high response rate is critical to success in assessing a culture, and a team training session has a committed, multidisciplinary audience that can ensure effective survey administration. As culture lives at a unit level, the ability to respectfully reflect the perceptions of various caregiver types is a powerful device to drive behavioral change.

At the beginning of the training session, to help draw in providers, you may want to use a story to encourage their participation and make the topic "real." Throughout the training you should focus on what their perceptions of teamwork are and how observations of their environment show a different story (*see* Chapter 7 for more information on observing teamwork and communication).

To be successful, these training sessions should have ALL members of the care team present, including physicians. Those organizations serious about enhancing teamwork and communication make it mandatory for everyone to attend. In organizations where physicians are employees, making teamwork training sessions mandatory is fairly straightforward. Those organizations with licensed independent practitioners may have more of a challenge, but creative approaches can help solicit physician participation. For example, one organization offered a stipend for every physician who practices in the hospital to attend team training. The hospital was then able to make attendance mandatory. Another hospital tied participation in teamwork training to the credentialing process and made it a requirement for physicians to attend. Involving physicians in team training can be challenging, but if you don't involve them, then all the teamwork training in the world will not enhance the dynamics of the care team and improve safety.

REFERENCES

1. Reinertsen JL. Zen and the art of physician autonomy maintenance. *Ann Intern Med.* 2003 Jun 17;138(12):992–995.
2. Bosk CL. *Forgive and Remember: Managing Medical Failure.* Chicago: University of Chicago Press, 1979.
3. Leonard MW, Frankel AS. Role of effective teamwork and communication in delivering safe, high-quality care. *Mt Sinai J Med.* 2011;78(6):820–826.
4. Detert JR, Edmondson AC. Everyday failures in organizational learning: Explaining the high threshold for speaking up at work (Harvard Business School Faculty Working Papers). Cambridge, MA, Oct 2006. Accessed Oct 31, 2012. http://community.psion.com/cfs-filesystemfile.ashx/__key/communityserver-blogs-components-weblogfiles/00-00-00-00-25/8836.Explaining-the-high-treshold-for-speaking-up-at-work.pdf
5. Leonard M, Frankel A, Simmonds T, editors: *Achieving Safe and Reliable Healthcare: Strategies and Solutions.* Chicago: Health Administration Press, 2004.
6. Schein EH. *Helping: How to Offer, Give and Receive Help.* San Francisco: Berrett-Koehler, 2009.
7. The Joint Commission. Behaviors That Undermine a Culture of Safety. *Sentinel Event Alert* No. 40. Jul 9, 2008. Accessed Oct 31 2012. http://www.jointcommission.org/sentinel_event_alert_issue_40_behaviors_that_undermine_a_culture_of_safety/.
8. Edmondson AC, Bohmer R, Pisano GP. Speeding up team learning. *Harv Bus Rev.* 2001;79(9):125–134.
9. Edmondson AC. *Teaming: How Organizations Learn, Innovate, and Compete in the Knowledge Economy.* San Francisco: Jossey-Bass, 2012.
10. Mazzocco K, et al. Surgical team behaviors and patient outcomes. *Am J Surg.* 2009;197(5):678–685.
11. Edmondson AC. Managing the risk of learning: Psychological safety in work teams. In West M, Tjosvold D, Smith K, editors: *International Handbook of Organizational Teamwork and Cooperative Working.* Hoboken, NJ: Wiley, 2003, 255–275.
12. Rosenstein AH, Russell H, Lauve R. Disruptive physician behavior contributes to nursing shortage. *Physician Exec.* 2002;28(6):8–11.
13. Makary MA, et al. Operating room briefings: Working on the same page. *Jt Comm J Qual Patient Saf.* 2006;32(6):351–355.
14. Leonard MW, Frankel AS. How can leaders influence a culture of safety? (Health Foundation Position Paper). London: May 2012. Accessed Oct 31, 2012. http://www.health.org.uk/publications/how-can-leaders-influence-a-safety-culture/#.
15. Helmreich RL, Merritt AC. *Culture at Work in Aviation and Medicine: National, Organizational and Professional Influences.* Aldershot, UK: Ashgate Press, 1998.
16. World Health Organization (WHO). *WHO Guidelines for Safe Surgery 2009: Safe Surgery Saves Lives.* Geneva: WHO, 2009. Accessed Oct 31, 2012. http://www.who.int/patientsafety/safesurgery/tools_resources/9789241598552/en/.
17. The High 5s Project. Home page. Accessed Oct 31, 2012. https://www.high5s.org/bin/view/Main/WebHome.
18. Haynes AB, et al. A surgical safety checklist to reduce morbidity and mortality in a global population. *N Engl J Med.* 2009 Jan 29;360(5):491–499.
19. van Klei WA, et al. Effects of the introduction of the WHO "Surgical Safety Checklist" on in-hospital mortality: A cohort study. *Ann Surg.* 2012;255(1):44–49.
20. de Vries EN, et al. Effect of a comprehensive surgical safety system on patient outcomes. *N Engl J Med.* 2010 Nov 11;363(20):1928–1937.
21. Personal communication between the author [M.L.] and Marja A. Boermeester, MD, Associate Professor, Department of Surgery, Academic Medical Centre, Amsterdam, Nov 27, 2011.
22. University Medical Center Groningen. Reduced risk of prosthetic infections thanks to behavioral and technical measures taken in operating room (online; no longer available). Groningen, Netherlands.
23. Timmel J, et al. Impact of the Comprehensive Unit-based Safety Program (CUSP) on safety culture in a surgical inpatient unit. *Jt Comm J Qual Patient Saf.* 2010 Jun;36(6):252–260.
24. The Joint Commission. Sentinel Event Data—Root Causes by Event Type: 2004–2Q 2012. Oct 18, 2012. Accessed Oct 31, 2012. http://www.jointcommission.org/Sentinel_Event_Statistics/.
25. The Joint Commission. *2012 Comprehensive Accreditation Manual for Hospitals: The Official Handbook.* Oak Brook, IL: Joint Commission Resources, 2011.
26. Biller CK, et al. The 80-hour work guidelines and resident survey perceptions of quality. *J Surg Res.* 2006;135(2):275–281.
27. Accreditation Council for Graduate Medical Education. Common Program Requirements. Jul 1, 2011. Accessed Oct 31, 2012. http://www.acgme-2010standards.org/pdf/Common_Program_Requirements_07012011.pdf.
28. Bandari J, et al. Surfacing safety hazards using standardized operating room briefings and debriefings at a large regional medical center. *Jt Comm J Qual Patient Saf.* 2012;38(4):154–160.

29. Haig KM, Sutton S, Whittington J. SBAR: A shared mental model for improving communication between clinicians. *Jt Comm J Qual Patient Saf.* 2006;32(3):167–175.

30. Macones GA, et al. The 2008 National Institute of Child Health and Human Development workshop report on electronic fetal monitoring: Update on definitions, interpretation, and research guidelines. *Obstet Gynecol.* 2008;112(3):661–666.

31. Klein G. *Sources of Power: How People Make Decisions.* Cambridge, MA: MIT Press, 1999.

32. Preston P. Learning from human factors: Getting it right in perinatal care. Paper presented at the Kaiser Permanente Partnership for Perinatal Patient Safety Conference, San Francisco, Oct 2003.

33. Stone D, Patton B, Heen S. *Difficult Conversations: How to Discuss What Matters Most.* New York: City Penguin Books, 1999.

34. Sexton JB, et al. The Safety Attitudes Questionnaire: Psychometric properties, benchmarking data, and emerging research. *BMC Health Serv Res.* 2006 Apr 3;6:44.

35. Salas E, et al. Does crew resource management training work? An update, an extension and some critical needs. *Hum Factors.* 2006;48(2):392–412.

36. Zwarenstein M, et al. Interprofessional education: Effects on professional practice and health care outcomes. *Cochrane Database Syst Rev.* 2001;(1):CD002213.

Chapter Seven

USING DIRECT OBSERVATION AND FEEDBACK TO MONITOR TEAM PERFORMANCE

Allan Frankel, MD; Andrew P. Knight, PhD

As discussed in Chapter 6, to improve performance of teams you must engage them in comprehensive and regular team training, which involves teaching communication strategies and skills, fostering interactions, engaging in role play, and practice, practice, practice.

A critical part of all change processes is measuring whether change has an effect, and so too, in efforts to improve teamwork the first question to ask, before asking about changes in clinical outcomes, is whether team training changes team behaviors. A common error is to focus immediately on whether the team training will affect the work produced by the team. Ultimately that is the goal, although in reality teamwork should affect three aspects of the team—the work produced, the satisfaction derived from the team in performing that work, and the ability of the team to improve itself. Knowing first whether team training has had an effect, and secondarily whether team work output has changed, allows the two measurements to be related to each other and provides a reasonable degree of evidence that change in one influences the other.

One measure of team practice is whether the individuals who comprise the team perform the agreed-on team behaviors and manifest the team norms of conduct. Careful observations of these behaviors can be compared against team performance and adverse outcome rates (if measurable). Historically, this type of observation has tended to be performed in research settings using researchers who spend significant effort to learn the fundamentals of social psychology followed by extensive training in observation. The authors of this book have moved from the perspective that observation is a research tool to a reframed perspective that

observation should be feasible as a quality assessment tool. Frontline clinicians with some clinical expertise and careful training can observe team behaviors in real time and evaluate how teammates interact with one another, and how well they work together toward a common goal. Careful and focused training is making this a reality.

There are fundamental and definable components of assessing the effectiveness of interventions aimed at improving team skills. This type of data collection involves observing the essential characteristics of team behavior and leadership in a way that is accurate and reproducible.

People, in general, are sensitive social instruments, and each of us is naturally quite good at evaluating social environments, as evidenced by immediate awareness of the tension level or feeling of comfort that exists in a room when we walk into social situations. This applies to trained observers who can evaluate with reasonable reliability three characteristics of a clinical environment[1]:

1. Observers can note the physical characteristics that might increase risk, from something as obvious as wires or tubing on a floor presenting a tripping hazard to incomplete patient information in a chart.

2. Observers can objectively and reproducibly observe specific defined behaviors, which will be discussed below.

3. Observers may characterize leaders and their ability to support team function.

It is important to note what observers cannot see. Observers cannot observe how team members feel or their attitudes or perceptions about the work environment. They can merely observe behaviors, actions, and the environment itself. Culture surveys, which are intended to capture team members' self-reported perceptions and attitudes, provide a different and equally important lens on the work environment.

As discussed in Chapter 2, the evaluation of culture, sometimes called climate, is perceived as an increasingly important component of improving the safety and reliability of health care organizations. For example, The Joint Commission requires that all hospitals perform safety culture surveys: Leadership Standard LD.03.01.01, "Leaders create and maintain a culture of safety and quality throughout the hospital," Element of Performance 1, "Leaders regularly evaluate the culture of safety and quality using valid and reliable tools."[2] Culture surveys, which can realistically be performed about every year, provide a snapshot of attitudes, which combined produce the organization's culture.

Observation is another measurement of culture, and as both attitudinal survey measures and behavioral observation measures become better understood and refined, they will give overlapping images of the environment of care in which providers function.

In clinical settings from ICUs to operating rooms (ORs) where teams do physical interventions and there is enough person-to-person interaction to make for a rich observation climate, it is feasible to link direct observation to an organization's safety culture survey.

Observation is based on a more objective perspective of culture, and multiple small observations, done serially over time, may offer a dynamic view of behavior. Senior leadership should look closely at these two types of data to get a picture of the safety and teamwork culture of different units within the organization.

The evidence for linking provider attitude and behaviors to real clinical outcomes is becoming increasingly persuasive, as evidenced by the Keystone project in Michigan, where the most successful ICUs that achieved the lowest bloodstream infections secondary to central line placement were also the ICUs with the highest scores in teamwork.[3] In Kaiser Permanente, Southern California Region, hospitals' teamwork behaviors—information sharing during intraoperative phases, briefing during handoff phases, and information sharing during handoff phases—were linked to decreased postoperative complications.[4] These studies and others are generating a solid body of evidence to support the logic of monitoring and measuring attitude and behaviors and applying teamwork programs to improve them.[5]

HOW TO USE DIRECT OBSERVATION

Although nonmedical industries employ observation to monitor and improve team processes and communication, the "gold standard" method for doing so in health care has yet to fully emerge but is well on its way.[6,7] To effectively observe team performance, you must have a systematic process in which trained observers measure performance using standardized definitions. When incorporating a systematic process for observation into your organization, consider the following points:

• How many observations should you do? How frequently? This will depend on the number of teams you are observing and the amount of data you want to collect. Formal observations of interventional areas require ongoing observation. One way to do this is to use sampling methods, such as a minimum of 5 observations per month—ideally, 10 to 15. These should be 30-minute observations and can occur in areas such as ORs, obstetric cesarean-section suites, interventional radiology suites, and gastroenterology suites.

Another option would be to concentrate observations during a two-month period and then repeat the observations some months later. However, the "right" number of observations done in this way has yet to be ascertained from current research. One large, academic interventional radiology department ultimately found that, from a practical standpoint in terms of time expenditure and the ability to implement observation, performing concentrated observations every three months was the most effective approach. In this case, the organization kept the size of its observer-trained group between 10 and 20 and asked each observer to perform 10 30-minute observations in a period of a few weeks near the end of each quarter. The end result was somewhere between 100 and 200 observations every three months. Because observations were performed during a concentrated period of time, this approach allowed the entire department to briefly adjust schedules to facilitate the observations.[8]

• When should you observe? It is helpful to assess team performance both before and after team training. Observation efforts before team training can highlight differences between team members' perception of their behavior and reality. It can reveal areas of risk and opportunities for improvement. By sharing these differences with team members during team training programs, you can clearly illustrate the current picture and where the team needs to improve. This can encourage buy-in and participation in team training as well as awareness of the work that needs to be done.

Assessing team performance after team training helps measure the effect of training on the behaviors and efforts of the team. Are there differences in performance? Observing after team training can also help identify where posttraining efforts should focus. For example, teams may be doing reasonable briefings and time-outs but few end-of-process debriefings, in which case this important team behavior can be made a topic for further discussion by the unit.

• What should you observe? As mentioned above, observers are able to characterize environmental threats; specific team behaviors, such as briefings, read-backs, callouts, time-outs, and Situation, Background, Assessment, Recommendation (SBAR)[9]; and leadership characteristics, such as motivating the team, seeking input, and resolving conflict. (*See* Sidebar 7-1 on page 72 for a more complete list.) Organizations can observe any or all of these; however, if you consider your observers to be like laboratory instruments, they understandably have capacity limits, and if used inappropriately will generate poor data. The key in observation is understanding the skills and limitations of your instruments (the observers), and designing observation methods to enhance interrater reliability while at the same time generating data that will be useful to the observed units and frontline providers.

Some behaviors are easy to evaluate, others are more subtle. Some behaviors occur infrequently, making it unlikely that observers will see them during their observation period. The two behaviors most easily observed are briefings and debriefings,[10] described in detailed in Chapter 6. During these team events, observers have the opportunity to observe multiple aspects of teamwork, leadership, and learning.

Briefings can be graded on the degree to which goals and the game plan are articulated; however, note that observers will have a harder time evaluating the degree to which each team member understands the goals and game plan because there are unlikely to be significant observable clues about their understanding unless team members are specifically asked to articulate the goals and game plan. Other aspects of briefings that are observable are the degree to which team members are reminded and assured of psychological safety and the importance of speaking up about

concerns; whether any specific team behaviors are identified during the briefings; and, finally, whether expectations of excellence are described. These together are the basic components of an effective briefing, and each is observable.

Debriefings are observable and can be graded based on whether the appropriate questions are asked—beginning with the basic ones of "What did we do well?" "What didn't we do well?" "What would we like to do differently?" Other important aspects of debriefings include whether all team members actively participate in the debriefing; whether the information elicited is documented on paper or some other recording mechanism: and the order of who speaks and the degree of psychological safety that appears to exist during the debriefing.

• How elegantly you define and describe what observers should look at makes an impact on how accurate their observations are. For example, good teams manifest situational awareness—knowing one's own actions relative to the whole, and, concurrently, being aware of the actions of others. Asking observers to evaluate situational awareness is tricky because, while there are some actions that might clue in the observer, situational awareness is a mind-set, and not necessarily observable. Make sure items are clearly defined to prevent confusion and problems with consistency. A proxy for situational awareness is offering help. If situational awareness and offering help are both on an observation sheet, it's unlikely that observers will be able to differentiate the one from the other.

• How should you observe? There are two primary ways of observing:

1. The checklist method. With this method, observers stand in the unit or patient care area and note the performance of team behaviors, such as read-backs, debriefings, and callouts. They look for whether the behaviors occur at the required or expected time (per observer evaluation), and they give each behavior a grade depending on how well the behavior was performed. When finished, observers can count the frequency of a behavior and assign a grade to the behavior by taking an average of the individual scores.

2. The gestalt method. This is akin to watching a sports team play a game and then assessing at the end how well the team played overall and performed the various functions that make up the sport. With this method, observers familiarize themselves with the behavioral metrics just before entering the clinical setting and then enter a unit for about

---

Sidebar 7-1. Behaviors Observed Using the CATS Tool

Following are the types of behaviors observed using the Communication and Teamwork Skills (CATS) tool. Three behaviors were identified as not consistently applicable in routine, noncrisis situations—"establishing an event manager," "escalation of asserted concern," and "critical language." These behaviors were positioned at the bottom of the CATS tool for use during critical events or if a routine event became critical.

- *Briefing:* This is a conversation and two-way dialogue of concise and relevant information shared prior to a procedure or activity.
- *Verbalize plan:* Speak aloud the next steps for the procedure and/or care of the patient.
- *Verbalize expected time frames:* Speak aloud time frames for particular interventions. "We'll give this another two minutes and if there's no change we'll try X."
- *Debriefing:* A conversation and two-way dialogue of concise and relevant information shared after the procedure or activity is completed.
- *Establish event manager if crisis arises:* Verbally identify who's in charge if situation becomes a crisis; event manager does not participate in active interventions but maintains situational awareness and verbalizes plans, needs, and time frames.
- *Visually scan environment:* Clinicians look up, look at one another, look at equipment, and look around the room.
- *Verbalize adjustments in plan as changes occur:* Speak aloud new plans, changes in strategy or intervention, and new time lines as procedure progresses.
- *Request additional external resources if needed:* Speak aloud, asking for help from outside the team—other clinicians, rooms, equipment, consults, and so forth.
- *Ask for help from team as needed:* Team members speak aloud, asking for assistance from members of the team.
- *Verbally request team input:* Ask aloud for team's suggestions, opinions, comments, or ideas.

- *Cross-monitoring:* Acknowledge concerns of others—watching team members, awareness of their actions, verbally stating concerns, sharing workload, verbally updating others in a manner less formal than briefing, responding to the concerns of team members.
- *Speak up, verbal assertion:* If team members are uncomfortable or unclear, they speak aloud their concerns and state an alternative viewpoint or suggest an alternative course of action. Individuals are sufficiently persistent to clearly state their opinions. If team members perceive something as unsafe, they speak aloud to indicate that. If responses to expressed concerns are not satisfactory and unsafe situations continue, individuals escalate the concern by bringing in other clinicians.
- *Closed-loop communication:* When a request is made of team members, someone specifically affirms aloud that they will complete the task and states aloud when the task has been completed.
- *SBAR:* Use of specific structured communication that states the situation, background, assessment, and recommendation.
- *Critical language:* Use of key phrases understood by all team members to mean "stop and listen; we have a potential problem." Specific phrases may differ from one institution or work unit to another.
- *Verbal updates of situation:* Think aloud—Team members verbally state their perceptions, actions, and plans as the procedure progresses.
- *Use team members' names:* Use team members' names.
- *Communicate with patient:* Team members speak to and respond to the patient.
- *Use appropriate tone of voice:* Team members use a tone of voice that is calm, professional, and not unnecessarily loud.

Source: Frankel A, et al. Using the Communication and Teamwork Skills (CATS) Assessment to measure health care team performance. *Jt Comm J Qual Patient Saf.* 2007;33(9):549–558.

---

20 minutes and watch the provision of care. They then leave and, looking at the list of metrics, identify what behaviors they saw. They grade those behaviors in overview, summing mentally all the individual episodes into one and using a predetermined Likert scale. Interestingly enough, a trained observer can do just as good a job at scoring using the gestalt method as the checklist method.

- Who is going to conduct the observations? The simplest answer to this question is either domain experts or others. Domain experts—those individuals who work in the

environment every day—will be more sensitive to the nuances of teamwork and communication behaviors but will be less objective. This is their department and their coworkers, and their perceptions of people are going to have inherent bias. On the good side, they will pick up subtle cues that a nondepartment member will miss, and they will understand clinical context, which is key to understanding complex relationships. However, they will also be accustomed to the status quo and desensitized to possibly glaring deficits. Consequently, you may opt, instead, to bring observers in from outside to do the observations. Although outside observers are more objective, they will be less sensitive, missing some of the issues and interactions that are more subtle.

To overcome the liabilities of both domain experts and outside observers, you may choose to use both types of observers, which can help ensure that the observation is accurate, but may influence the rating reliability. Our experience suggests that the interrater reliability degradation is not that significant. What also tends to happen is that when the two types of observers are trained together, they tend to benefit from understanding each other's point of view. Often the greatest discrepancies between observers when they initially train together are the different perspectives on and awareness of patient involvement, clinician-patient interactions, and the teamwork process. Whether domain experts or others, some observers are very aware of how patients are engaged in the team dynamics, while others overlook the interactions with patients—until the topic is broached in training. It is essential that domain experts and outsider observers have a common definition and understanding of the behaviors that the department perceives as important.

• How are you going to score the observations? Defining a consistent scoring system is critical to ensure observers rate performance reliably. Be realistic. Observers that are not so sensitive that they will reliably give the same scores across a 10-point scale, ranging from excellent to poor team behaviors. In truth, a 10-point scale is unnecessary to direct efforts to improve teamwork. Observers appear to do well when asked to characterize behaviors on a 4- or 5-point scale of unacceptable, poor, adequate, good, and excellent. Remember the purpose of observations—to identify those behaviors amenable to improvement, and to highlight those done well. A 4-point scale is adequate for this task.

• How are you going to train observers? Effective, comprehensive, and consistent training is key to achieving success with this data collection method. Observers must be trained in groups so that they can learn from each other.

One option for training involves using standardized videos of different scenarios, which are shown to groups who then score them, debrief, and compare their scores. Significant score differences are discussed so that varying points of view are highlighted. The videos are played over

again, sometimes multiple times, to help the group develop standardized ways of looking at behaviors. In the process, individual observers become sensitized to their biases and instructed to keep these in mind when scoring. For example, some observers set unrealistic expectations for themselves and project those expectations onto those they observe. When their scores are lower than the rest of the training group, they are forced to reflect on their bias and adjust.

Occasionally, some individuals are attuned to the social environment so differently that they are unable to come in line with the observer group, and it is reasonable to not use these individuals as observers. Some of us do see things differently! Showing all observers a standardized set of videos enables everyone to receive the same training on what to observe, how to observe, and how to score what is observed. Although organizations may need to devote several days to this training to ensure that observers are trained thoroughly and appropriately, we have had success in training groups of domain experts and nonclinicians in about half a day—if the training is well orchestrated and efficient.

Departments that have continued conducting observations for a period of time realize the importance of periodically—usually, about every three months—bringing the observers together for an hour or 90-minute "recalibration" meeting. This time together is an opportunity to do a variety of things. For example, observers can raise issues of concern or bring up situations they have run into during previous observations that have been problematic or particularly useful learning experiences. Often, the observers describe how these recalibration meetings are useful in reminding them about the components that generally predispose operational excellence and therefore put into context the observation process. A common discussion during these periods is the inevitable evolution of observers from purely measures of behavior to coaches of the team. This change is profound. It means that the observation process becomes less one of auditing and more one of teaching, and it suggests that the team members develop a greater appreciation of the team behaviors. Observers are often nurses or technicians, so their role changes significantly as they develop the skill to coach teams whose participants will often include physicians. This transformation, overall, is a healthy one because it indicates greater appreciation and acceptance of the importance of teamwork and moves the responsibility for the teamwork behaviors squarely onto the team members themselves. Good observers learn to ask nonjudgmental questions and link the team behaviors to advantages for staff and patients and thereby decrease team members' defensiveness and perception of criticism. Ultimately, the observers become embedded and real champions for effective teamwork and culture.

• How are you going to ensure interrater reliability? In the context of observation, interrater reliability is the level of agreement between two observers. When interrater reliability is good, two observers will grade team performance in a similar way. When it is not good, observers will vary in their grading, skewing the results and degrading measurement accuracy. It is important to both establish and maintain interrater reliability. Good training is key to establishing such reliability. According to Landis and Koch, values for kappa, the statistic indicating the strength of agreement,[11] can be classified as poor (< 0.00), slight (0.00–0.20), fair (0.21–0.40), moderate (0.41–0.60), substantial (0.61–0.80), and almost perfect (0.81–1.00).[12]

To maintain reliability, observers must perform paired observations during which they will need to follow a stricter set of rules than in normal observations. A simple example explains why. If two observers enter an OR and move to separate parts of the room, or even stand side by side but see different parts of the room, then they are likely to observe different sets of interactions. One might see the anesthesiologist in discussion with a nurse, while the other may see the surgeon and scrub technician speaking to each other. If the two observers compare notes afterward they will have seen different parts of the procedure, and their results will be different. Observers testing interrater reliability should agree to focus on similar team actions and then discuss only those activities.

Standardizing the Scoring of Behaviors

Regardless of the observation model your organization uses, a key challenge is achieving interrater reliability among the observers. As mentioned earlier, a mainstay of observer training is to show videos that illustrate a variety of teamwork behaviors and then discuss observer perceptions. This educational process is enhanced when observers have a set of definitions that reflect both excellent and poor team behaviors. Table 7-1 (pages 75–77) includes both definitions and examples. This type of table is quite beneficial in observation training.

• How are you going to analyze data collected during observation? Turning completed observation sheets into simply understandable reports is key. The two characteristics that can be documented for each observed metric are frequency and quality. While quality is always important, the utility of frequency varies. For example, when observing the beginning of a procedure, it is probably reasonable to expect that a briefing will be observed and scored. If no briefing occurs, that is significant. If a briefing is seen, identifying its quality is the next measurement.

On the other hand, most units would be deeply troubled to see a conflict resolution score on every observation sheet, regardless of the quality, as that would imply that conflict was an endemic characteristic of the unit. Equally troublesome, however, is periodic scoring of unresolved conflict, indicating that while the team generally gets along well, when it doesn't, it lacks the skills to address the issues.

• How are you going to share data with patient care teams and leaders? Sharing information is a key component to getting buy-in for improvement efforts and for giving feedback when improvement efforts are under way. By graphically displaying the different spectrum of scores, you can visually communicate the effectiveness of team performance and areas of improvement. This can provide motivation for improvement and reinforce desired behaviors.

METHODS OF DIRECT OBSERVATION

The following sections discuss two current models for direct observation.

The TICOT Model for Direct Observation

Building on research models from crisis resource management and applying insights from the social and cognitive psychology literature, the Teamwork in Context Observation Tool (TICOT) model is used to evaluate threats, team behaviors, team relationships, and leadership characteristics in interventional teams. The one-page metric is designed to address three conflicting tensions: the ability of human beings to observe and characterize social events; the limits of the human mind to track multiple variables at one time; and the desire to keep observation as a simple tool for quality evaluations, affordable in the health care climate.

As mentioned earlier, humans are thoroughly social beings with sensitized antennae for how individuals interact

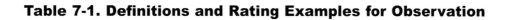

Table 7-1. Definitions and Rating Examples for Observation

Item	Definition	Rating = 1 Examples	Rating = 2 Examples	Rating = 3 Examples	Rating = 4 Examples
1. The physical environment supported safe care.	Lighting, ergonomics, tripping hazards (for example, cords), temperature, noise, etc., facilitate safe treatment of patient(s).	• Construction noise makes it hard to hear. • Lighting is very dim making it hard to see.	• Multiple people comment on it being too hot or too cold. • Room is disorganized.	• Room is clean, orderly, and ergonomically designed. • Room is well-lit.	• Room is spotless and exceptionally organized. • Team members positively note the room.
2. Equipment and materials were available and worked well.	All needed clinical and operational equipment and materials are immediately at-hand and functions as expected.	• Team members are unable to access a piece of needed equipment. • Equipment breaks down.	• Delay(s) in accessing equipment • Equipment functionality is patchy/spotty.	• No need to ask for additional equipment. • All equipment functions as expected.	• In unexpected situation, extra equipment is accessed without delay and functions well.
3. Expertise not in the team was effectively accessed when needed.	When outside clinical, technical, or other experts are required to facilitate patient care, these individuals are quickly and easily accessed.	• Unable to access critical, needed expertise. • "Expert" does not possess expertise.	• Delay occurs accessing or identifying expertise. • Difficulty communicating with external expertise.	• Expertise is available and quickly accessed. • Flow of patient care is hardly interrupted.	• In unexpected situation, expert integrates seamlessly into the team. • Communication flawless.
4. All the necessary information for diagnostic and therapeutic decisions (for example, history, labs, test) was available when needed.	Specific pieces of clinical information such as patient history, lab results, and test results are at-hand and accessed in a quick and easy manner.	• Unable to access critical, needed information. • Request for information is refused or rejected.	• Significant delay in accessing information. • Difficulty in interpreting/reading information.	• Information is available and quickly accessed. • Flow of patient care is hardly interrupted.	• In unexpected situation, information is rapidly accessed and integrated to inform team plan.
5. Interruptions and distractions were well-managed.	Telephone calls, irrelevant conversations, and comments are kept to a minimum. Any unavoidable interruptions are handled effectively.	• Irrelevant interruptions distract from team tasks. • Other interruptions overwhelm the team.	• Irrelevant interruptions delay task completion. • Other interruptions lead to significant delays.	• Irrelevant interruptions are quickly dismissed. • Other interruptions are quickly built into the plan.	• High volume of unavoidable interruptions are managed and built into team plan.
6. Staffing was sufficient to handle the workload.	The quantity and variety of task personnel are adequate for effectively performing tasks.	• Personnel are absent or unavailable, resulting in delays, cancellations, or increased risk.	• The team appears to struggle with workload due to insufficient personnel.	• Staffing is adequate for effective performance of team tasks.	• When work pace / volume increases, staffing rises accordingly to meet new needs.
7. Team members worked together as a well-coordinated team.	Team interactions are seamless and flow with minimal confusion. The team effectively transitions across changing circumstances and task requirements.	• Significant confusion interrupts team tasks. • Risk increases due to bungled interactions.	• The team is confused and regroups frequently. • Interactions appear clumsy or ineffective.	• Interactions are seamless and flow with little confusion. • Transitions are smooth.	• In the face of unexpected situations the team coordination remains seamless.
8. Team members treated one another with respect.	All members of the team interact with one another in a polite, professional, and courteous manner, showing regard for each team member's role.	• Members devalue others explicitly. • There is a clear and explicit lack of respect.	• One or more members is talked down to at times. • Team members are implicitly devalued.	• All interactions are polite, professional, and courteous. • Team is appropriately engaged in the tasks.	• The importance of all team member roles for the team's success is explicitly stated.
9. Situational awareness was maintained (for example, task prioritization and awareness of red flag issues).	Team members are aware of their surroundings and cognizant of increased risk levels generated by specific practices and actions.	• People are absent-minded, preoccupied, or overwhelmed. • Critical risks are missed.	• People are on "auto-pilot" and not fully engaged in tasks. • Team is lackadaisical.	• Team focus increases as tasks warrant.	• As unexpected circumstances arise, they are verbally noted and clearly organized.
10. Important issues were well-communicated at handoffs (for example, shift changes, patient transfers).	When responsibility for care changes providers or teams, information is communicated in a structured manner (*see* SBAR below).	• Handoffs occur without information exchange. • Handoffs are done implicitly.	• Information exchange is unstructured at handoffs. • Handoff is rushed and/or incomplete.	• Information exchange is structured at handoff. • Complete information needed for care given.	• Info exchange structured • Risk of handoff explicitly stated to raise attention during info exchange.

Table 7-1. Definitions and Rating Examples for Observation (continued)

Item	Definition	Rating = 1 Examples	Rating = 2 Examples	Rating = 3 Examples	Rating = 4 Examples
11. Disagreements were openly discussed until resolved in the patient's best interest.	Points of contention or differences of opinion are brought out in the open and discussed with the patient's interests as the goal of resolution.	• Disagreements erupt into hot exchanges. • Team members lose tempers.	• Disagreements are not discussed. • Disagreements focus on "who is wrong."	• Differences lead to critical thinking. • Focus of discussion is patient's best interests.	• When appropriate, differences of opinion yield learning for one or more members.
12. Briefing and rebriefing	Formal task/actions briefing occurs at the start of a procedure. Formal / distinct re-briefing occurs when conditions change in the midst of a procedure.	• Formal briefing does not occur when appropriate (for example, start of procedure). • Lack of game plan and discussions lead to increased risk.	• Formal briefing is disorganized. • Components of formal briefing are incomplete. • Game plan is not always clear to all.	• Names/roles and procedure verified. • All know the game plan. • Details, critical steps, and possible problems raised and readdressed.	• Importance of briefing for effective performance/ communication emphasized. • All know the game plan all the time.
13. Sharing information	Information is offered and received both formally and informally as team members speak up with observations, recommendations, and intentions.	• Sharing is discouraged (for example, "keep quiet"). • Sharing doesn't occur when it should.	• Shared info is ignored or glossed over. • Sharing of info is too quiet and/or passive.	• Info sharing is met with engagement by others. • Info is shared overtly and with confidence.	• Importance of sharing info is emphasized by team members. • Thanks given for sharing.
14. Asking for information	Information is sought both formally and informally as team members ask questions for clarification from others to resolve ambiguities.	• Those asking for info are made to feel stupid. • Those who seem unsure fail to ask questions.	• Requests for info are ignored or glossed over. • Requests for info are too quiet and/or passive.	• Requests for info are met with engagement and clear responses. • Ambiguities are resolved.	• Requests for info are met with engagement. • Requests are welcomed, appreciated, or thanked.
15. Assertion and challenge	Members stand their ground when concerned about team actions or not in agreement with decision, challenging the team for clarification or consensus.	• Challenge discouraged. • Those who don't agree "go with the flow" without raising concerns.	• When challenge exhibited it is squashed. • Discomfort remains but the team proceeds.	• When challenge occurs, additional information is sought and obtained to inform team actions.	• Challenge yields more information being sought and is explicitly appreciated by team.
16. Structured communication (for example, SBAR)	Members use a formal communications protocol that structures information into the problem, the background, and an assessment and recommendation.	• Structured communication is not used. • Information is confused.	• Structured communication is inadequately used. • Structure is incorrect.	• Structured communication is used when pertinent. • Correct structure is used.	• In addition to using structured communication, members note its importance.
17. Closing the loop	Members confirm that information was received by repeating the content of the information back to the sender (that is, read-back and hear-back).	• Requests, orders, and instructions, rarely repeated, increase risk. • Information is confused.	• Requests, orders, and instructions are seldom repeated even though it is pertinent.	• Pertinent requests, orders, and instructions are repeated back to the sender when received.	• In addition to closing the loop, members note its importance.
18. Debriefing	Team conducts a formal debriefing covering what went well, what could be done better, and what might be improved and applied to future process.	• Debriefing does not occur when appropriate (for example, end of procedure).	• Debriefing does not cover relevant questions. • Debriefing does not yield clear takeaways.	• Debriefing held at end of procedure done correctly. • Debriefing generates clear takeaways.	• Debriefing exceptionally structured. • Members comment on importance of debriefing.
19. Leadership invited the input/feedback of others.	Team leaders explicitly ask team members to provide their thoughts, opinions, recommendations, and questions during team interactions.	• L-ship visibly reacts negatively to input. • L-ship explicitly dissuades input.	• L-ship does not explicitly invite input. • L-ship does not ask for feedback from team.	• L-ship explicitly asks the team for input. • L-ship invites all team member opinions.	• L-ship stresses the importance of member feedback for successful team functioning.

Table 7-1. Definitions and Rating Examples for Observation (continued)

Item	Definition	Rating = 1 Examples	Rating = 2 Examples	Rating = 3 Examples	Rating = 4 Examples
20. Leadership motivated the team to perform well.	Team leaders charge the team with their tasks and encourage high performance as a whole.	• L-ship hurts motivation with only neg. feedback. • L-ship devalues some team members.	• L-ship does not convene and engage whole team. • L-ship does not ask for high performance.	• L-ship convenes whole team and presents tasks. • L-ship asks for high collective performance.	• L-ship stresses value of teamwork. • L-ship expresses high expectations of team.
21. Leadership managed conflict.	Team leaders explicitly guide the resolution of conflict between team members and/or the leaders and team members.	• L-ship exacerbates conflict. • L-ship loses temper and/or control of team.	• L-ship fails to engage in managing conflict. • L-ship allows conflict to run on.	• L-ship guides discussion and resolution of conflict. • L-ship respects differences of members.	• L-ship uses conflict to spur learning. • L-ship revisits conflict when appropriate.

This table provides some key definitions and rating examples that can be used in observation training to enhance interrater reliability.

Source: Pascal Metrics, Inc. Used with permission.

with each other. However, like all quality instruments, humans must be focused in the right direction and periodically "recalibrated." Within the TICOT model, the questions asked of the observers are similar, and in some cases identical, to the questions on the Safety Attitudes Questionnaire discussed in Chapter 2. This was done to facilitate linking of the attitudinal survey scores with observed team behaviors and relationships. The TICOT model entails 21 observable metrics, with testing to date suggesting there is little overlap between the definitions, a key requirement to maintain interrater reliability. However, fine-tuning is necessary during observation training—for example, agreeing on the difference between briefings and sharing information. (A briefing is a more formal coming together of some of the or the entire group to ensure that the game plan is understood, while sharing information is less formal and may consist of only pieces of the whole game plan).

Finally, the TICOT model is designed to be completed after about a 20–40 minute observation period.

The TICOT questions are divided into four categories:
- Operational context
- Team climate and process
- Behaviors
- Leadership

Operational context evaluates the threats that, when evident, increase risk or decrease reliability of care. Observers are asked to rate the following statements[3]:

1. The physical environment supported safe care.

2. Equipment and materials were available and worked well.

3. Expertise not within the team was effectively accessed when needed.

4. All the necessary information for diagnostic and therapeutic decisions—history, labs, tests—was available when needed.

5. Interruptions and distractions were rare.

6. Staffing was sufficient to handle the workload.[4]

Team climate and process evaluates team member relationships using the following statements:

1. Team members worked together as a well-coordinated team.

2. Team members treated one another with respect.

3. Situational awareness was maintained (for example, there was task prioritization and awareness of red flag issues).

4. Important issues were well communicated at handoffs, such as during shift changes and patient transfers.

5. Disagreements were openly discussed until resolved in the patient's best interest.

Behaviors specific to good teamwork are evaluated by asking observers to rate the following:

1. Briefing and rebriefing

2. Sharing information

3. Asking for information

4. Assertion and challenge

5. Structured communication, such as SBAR

6. Closing the loop

7. Debriefing

Three essential leadership behaviors amenable to observation are as follows:

1. Leadership invited the input/feedback of others.

2. Leadership directed the team through its tasks.

3. Leadership managed conflict.

The 21 observable components are defined on the back of the metrics sheet, and observers are instructed to read the definitions before every observation to help ensure consistency in grading similar events.

As previously mentioned, careful collection of observed information is only the first part of turning observations into useful data. The presentation of the material is key to understanding and applying the findings in order to change and improve. Two aspects of observation data stand out. First is how frequently the 21 components are seen compared to the

observers' expectations. Second, when the behaviors are viewed, what is their quality? The most recent graphing of the data shows both components. (*See* Figure 7-1, below.)

The TICOT model works well, particulary in research. In general, departments that use the TICOT model for measuring the quality of teamwork tend to decrease the number of questions regarding the physical safety of the environment and a few team behaviors, such as briefing and debriefing.

The CATS Model

Variations of the Communication and Teamwork Skills (CATS) observation tool are in use in organizations around the country. Researchers at Partners Health Care developed this behavioral observation tool on the basis of principles of crisis resource management in nonmedical industries. The tool was designed to quantitatively assess communication and team skills of health care providers in a variety of real

Figure 7-1. Frequency and Quality of Observations

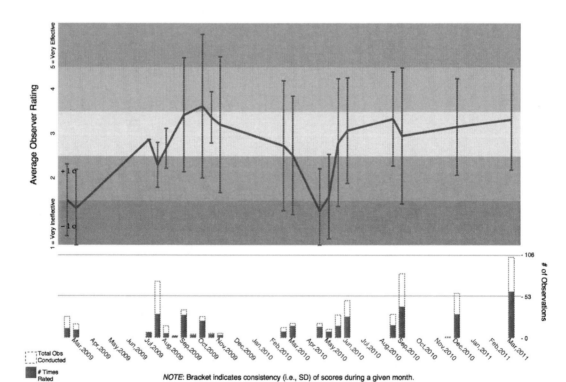

NOTE: Bracket indicates consistency (i.e., SD) of scores during a given month.

This figure presents a sample page displaying trend lines for the "behaviors" category in the TICOT model and includes how frequently behaviors were seen (the bars on the bottom) and the overall quality of the behaviors in the trend line.

Source: Pascal Metrics, Inc. Used with permission.

and simulated clinical settings.[13] Within this tool, specific behavior markers used for observation are clustered into the following four categories:

1. Coordination
2. Cooperation
3. Situational awareness
4. Communication

These four domains are subdivided into various elements, including the following:

- Planning and preparation
- Prioritization
- Execution
- Identifying and using resources
- Coordinating team activities
- Communicating and exchanging information

- Assertiveness and authority
- Assessing capabilities
- Supporting others
- Gathering information
- Understanding and recognition
- Anticipation
- Identifying options
- Balancing risks and selecting options
- Reevaluation

Teams are scored in terms of the occurrence and quality of specific behaviors during a routine or critical event. The scoring sheet (*see* Figure 7-2, below) is designed to allow the observer to mark each time that specific behaviors (*see* Sidebar 7-1 on page 72) occur and grade their quality. Three columns are provided for this:

Figure 7-2. CATS Observation Form

Category	Behaviors	Observed and Good	Variation in Quality	Expected but Not Observed
Coordination	Briefing			
	Verbalize plan			
	Verbalize expected time frames			
	Debriefing			
Awareness	Visually scan environment			
	Verbalize adjustments in plan as changes occur			
Cooperation	Request external resources if needed			
	Ask for help from team as needed			
	Verbally request team input			
	Cross-monitoring			
	Verbal assertion			
	Receptive to assertion and ideas			
Communication	Closed loop			
	SBAR			
	Verbal updates—think aloud			
	Use names			
	Communicate with patient			
	Appropriate tone of voice			

This scoring sheet is used to document the performance of observed behaviors.

Source: Partners Health Care, Inc. Used with permission.

1. "Observed and Good"

2. "Variation in Quality" (meaning incomplete or of variable quality)

3. "Expected but Not Observed"

Observers score behaviors on the degree to which the behavior meets a previously agreed-upon definition.

After each behavior is scored, a weighted total is obtained as follows:

- Marks in the "Observed and Good" column = 1

- Marks in the "Variation in Quality" column = .5

- Marks in the "Expected but Not Observed" column = 0

Scores are added together to achieve a weighted total. Thereafter, a second total is obtained by simply adding up the total number of marks made. The weighted total, divided by the total number of marks, adjusted to a 100-point scale, is the quality score for that behavior. In this manner, a quality score is established for each behavior during each observation period. Organizations using the CATS tool can then graphically display the different scores to show the current picture of teamwork, a comparison between pretraining and posttraining teams, and areas of improvement.

No matter which method of direct observation you use, measuring teamwork with a systematic process involving trained observers monitoring predefined team behaviors can help your organization get a realistic picture of how teamwork and communication occur on a particular unit.

REFERENCES

1. Yule S, et al. Surgeons' non-technical skills in the operating room: Reliability testing of the NOTSS behavior rating system. *World J Surg.* 2008;32(4):548–556.

2. The Joint Commission. *2012 Comprehensive Accreditation Manual for Hospitals: The Official Handbook.* Oak Brook, IL: Joint Commission Resources, 2011.

3. Rodriguez-Paz JM, Pronovost P. Prevention of catheter-related bloodstream infections. *Adv Surg.* 2008;42:229–248.

4. Mazzocco K, et al. Surgical team behaviors and patient outcomes. *Am J Surg.* 2009;197(5):678–685.

5. Garvin DA, Edmondson AC, Gino F. Is yours a learning organization? *Harv Bus Rev.* 2008;86(3):109–116, 134.

6. Groff H. Understanding CRICO's perinatal claims. *Forum.* 2001;21(1):1–14.

7. The Joint Commission. Preventing infant death and injury during delivery. *Sentinel Event Alert,* No. 30: Jul 21, 2004. Accessed Oct 31, 26, 2012. http://www.jointcommission.org/sentinel_event_alert_issue_30_preventing_infant_death_and_injury_during_delivery/.

8. Miguel K, Hirsch JA, Sheridan RM. Team training: A safer future for neurointerventional practice. *J Neurointerv Surg.* 2011;3(3):285–287.

9. Haig KM, Sutton S, Whittington J. SBAR: A shared mental model for improving communication between clinicians. *Jt Comm J Qual Patient Saf.* 2006;32(3):167–175.

10. Makary MA, et al. Operating room briefings: Working on the same page. *Jt Comm J Qual Patient Saf.* 2006;32(6):351–355.

11. Viera AJ, Garrett JM. Understanding interobserver agreement: The kappa statistic. *Fam Med.* 2005;37(5):360–363.

12. Landis JR, Koch GG. The measurement of observer agreement for categorical data. *Biometrics.* 1977;33(1):159–174.

13. Frankel A, et al. Using the Communication and Teamwork Skills (CATS) Assessment to measure health care team performance. *Jt Comm J Qual Patient Saf.* 2007;33(9):549–558.

Chapter Eight

DISCLOSURE

Doug Bonacum, MBA, BS; James Conway, MS; Douglas Salvador, MD, MPH

Despite the best of intentions and highly skilled caregivers, sometimes patients suffer inadvertent harm. A surgeon unintentionally nicks a patient's liver during a procedure. A patient has an unexpected heart attack during surgery. A patient is seriously injured after receiving the wrong dose of medication. A mix-up in drawing laboratory specimens leads to the patient's receiving the wrong blood, which triggers a fatal transfusion reaction. All these events are considered unanticipated, and every hospital in the country experiences them. An unanticipated outcome can be caused by many factors, including the following[1]:

- Inherent risks associated with an intervention
- Biologic variability—the confluence of rare and unavoidable circumstances
- The patient's condition
- Human error, either an act of omission or commission
- Drift from safe practice
- Breakdowns in communication, either between patient and practitioner(s), or among practitioner(s)
- Issues associated with clinical processes and treatment
- Malfunctions in a system used to provide care

While the previous chapters introduce the concept of systematically reducing risk and preventing errors from happening or preventing them from harming the patient, this chapter focuses on what to do when a medical error or other unanticipated event causes patient harm. Although the process of disclosure is similar for medical errors and other unanticipated events, different dynamics exist within the two scenarios: In the former, avoidable harm occurs related to the failure to deliver appropriate care, whereas in the latter, unanticipated events, either related to the patient's biologic variability or the care process, lead to an undesired outcome.

In addition to learning from the error or adverse event, organizations must be open and honest about what happened with patients, family, and the staff members involved. The process of telling the patient and family honestly what

happened, how it happened, and what's going to happen next is called disclosure. The word *disclosure* in legal terms may imply the release of protected information. The authors of *When Things Go Wrong: Responding to Adverse Events* prefer the term *communication,* to convey a sense of openness and reciprocity.[2]

DISCLOSING ADVERSE EVENTS

There are four main reasons why disclosing an adverse event is important:

1. It is the right thing to do. Patients and their families have a fundamental right to know what happened, how it happened, and how it can be prevented for the next patient. Consider if it were your family member. Wouldn't you want them to know what happened?

2. An adverse event has a huge lasting impact on everyone involved, and disclosure helps participants initiate the coping process. Open communication about an error helps patients and their families to understand why all outcomes cannot be anticipated and can reduce the patient and family's anger and frustration. This is essential to help rebuild trust. In addition, openly communicating about the situation may help a provider learn from the event and maintain a sense of personal and professional integrity. We often neglect the reality that health professionals are frequently the "second victim" of an adverse event.[3] Effective disclosure is an opportunity to reaffirm and build on the existing relationship between the care providers and the patient and his or her family.

3. By communicating openly about errors with patients and their families as well as with staff, you can identify and repair system issues that led to the error and identify opportunities for improvement.

4. Evidence from disclosure pioneers demonstrates that the public perception of an organization can improve if the organization engages in disclosure and suggests that disclosure

programs may not increase malpractice costs. The best example of highly effective patient-professional communication in response to disappointing outcomes is at the University of Michigan. As Kachalia et al. stated:

> After full implementation of a disclosure-with-offer program, the average monthly rate of new claims decreased from 7.03 to 4.52 per 100,000 patient encounters. . . . Average monthly cost rates decreased for total liability . . . patient compensation . . . and non–compensation-related legal costs.[4(p. 213)]

Yet the generalizability of these findings remains controversial. The Agency for Healthcare Research and Quality has funded at least four pilot programs in multicenter settings to provide more evidence for the outcomes of disclosure-with-offer (in which compensation is paid when the health care organization is at fault) programs.[5]

There is strong support for disclosure by health care professional societies, legislative bodies, and accreditation agencies. This support is consistent with a societal response to patient and family desires for transparency. Examples of this support include the following:

• Since 2003 The Joint Commission has required that patients and, when appropriate, their families be informed about the outcomes of care, including "unanticipated outcomes of care, treatment, and services" that have been provided.[6]

• In 2006 the National Quality Forum published a new safe-practice guideline on disclosure. It expects health care facilities to, "provide open and clear communication with patients and families regarding serious unanticipated outcomes."[7]

• The American Medical Association's Code of Medical Ethics includes the following statement: "Situations occasionally occur in which a patient suffers significant medical complications that may have resulted from the physician's mistake or judgment. In these situations, the physician is ethically required to inform the patient of all the facts necessary to ensure understanding of what has occurred."[8]

• In 2005 Lucian Leape led a group, which included individuals from the Harvard-affiliated hospitals and CRICO/Risk Management Foundation, as well as attorneys and patients, to develop a position paper grounded on two principles: Medical care must be safe and medical care must be patient centered. The authors state that ". . . the paper represents a moral argument, not a business case or evidence-based clinical guidelines." The authors continue: "This consensus paper of the Harvard-affiliated hospitals proposes a full disclosure when adverse events or medical errors occur, including an apology to the patient. The paper represents the collaborative effort of a group of clinicians, risk managers, and patients participating from several Harvard teaching hospitals and the Risk Management Foundation."[2] The paper was endorsed by the Harvard-affiliated institutions and CRICO/Risk Management Foundation.

• Disclosure policies are being formally adopted not only in the United States but across a range of countries, including Canada, Australia, New Zealand, and the United Kingdom.[9–11]

Barriers to Disclosure

Traditionally, health care organizations have shied away from disclosing adverse events to patients and their families for fear of lawsuits, inflammatory media reports, and bad publicity. Barriers to individual health care practitioners performing disclosure have been explored in surveys and focus studies.[12–14] Such barriers include the following:

• Fear of litigation

• Harm to reputation

• Discomfort with handling the emotional response of the patient and family

• Lack of training in communication

• Belief that patients and families are not capable of understanding the full complexity of events

• Uncertainty about which events to disclose

In a survey of 1,311 physicians and surgeons that asked what factors would make them less likely to disclose a serious error, 61% of the respondents felt that the patient would not understand the information; 27%, that the physician might get sued; 24%, that the patient was unaware of the error; and 19%, that the patient would not want to know about the error.[13] In addition to being afraid, providers who are involved with a medical mistake bring feelings of guilt, anxiety, and shame to the situation. Such feelings do not easily lend themselves to open and honest disclosure. The factors above must be considered when instituting an enterprisewide disclosure policy or assisting a physician in having a disclosure communication.

Overcoming the Fear of Litigation

When establishing strong commitment to and a process for disclosure, one of the most significant barriers your organization will need to overcome is the fear of being sued. Although there is evidence that suggests if you are open and honest with people around disclosure, you decrease the risk of malpractice, some providers are still hesitant. The fact is that people sue because there is a significant divergence between expectations and outcomes, and organizations don't manage that divergence effectively.[15–17] Given that the natural emotion associated with a bad outcome and inadequate disclosure/communication is anger, a goal to hurt the hospital or physician is typically the driving force toward litigation. It naturally follows then that providers who communicate openly, honestly, empathetically, and in a timely manner about the differences between expectations and outcomes will help reduce the likelihood of being sued.

Consider the following two examples: Several years ago, Abington Memorial Hospital—a 570-bed regional teaching hospital located in eastern Pennsylvania—treated an elderly gentleman, and, through a series of unfortunate diagnostic errors, inadvertently contributed to his death. Within the organization's quality assurance process, Abington discovered the error and determined that, although the family never questioned their loved one's death, the hospital felt obligated to disclose the missteps, which resulted in contributing to his untimely demise.

The treating physician and leaders from the organization visited the widow at her home and explained what happened, how it happened, and how very sorry they were. The patient's wife appreciated the organization's candor and responded by donating money to the organization to establish a memorial lectureship series in her husband's name at the hospital devoted to safety. Within this series, patient safety experts from around the country come to the hospital and speak about preventing error, creating a just culture, requiring open disclosure, and improving the quality and safety of the care they deliver. This also positively reinforces the prevailing safety culture of the hospital.

On the other side of the United States is a well-respected institution in which a 9-year-old girl with a highly curable form of acute leukemia entered the hospital for treatment. While in the hospital she developed a serious infection, which was not appropriately detected, and she died an avoidable death. Little explanation was provided to the family, and the organization has avoided the mother's pleas for information, despite multiple promises.

What does it say to this devastated family when they walk on the floor of the hospital where their child was a patient and no one will "look them in the eye"? The family, who went home without their child, will never be the same, and feels a profound lack of resolution and affirmation of their loss. The organization has clinicians who have been emotionally scarred by their involvement, and there is no open forum for learning, grieving, and improvement. The resident in charge of the girl's care was so upset that she quit her job.

Despite multiple interactions, the family does not believe that they have had the "right conversation" with the hospital. What does the family want—the truth, an apology, and someone to acknowledge there were lapses in care, and discuss what the organization has learned and done to prevent this tragic event from happening again. Nobody wins in this dynamic.

LEADERSHIP COMMITMENT TO DISCLOSURE IS CRITICAL

The board and senior leadership have the capacity to set an organizational expectation for honest, transparent, and effective patient-professional communication. Although their action is necessary, it is not sufficient for a successful program. This expectation must be accompanied by monitoring and follow-up to assess effectiveness. Leaders' actions that support disclosure include the following:

• Model organization values in times that are difficult. Disclosure conversations are never easy, and yet they are a clear sign of how much an organization's values are imbedded in the way it does business. Disclosure represents a true test of a culture in that it shows that the organization does the right thing even when it's not easy. The ability and willingness to do this sends important messages to the community and internally within the organization.

• Commit to a fair and just culture. (*See* Chapter 3 for more information.) Effective disclosure is dependent on a just culture. If a provider doesn't feel safe about speaking up about errors, there is little hope he or she will be comfortable sharing information with a patient.

• Be actively engaged in learning about adverse and potentially compensable events. What percentage of incidents resulting in medical malpractice claims and demand letters are you actively aware of and managing before they get to the point of legal action? The answer should be close to 100%; in many care systems it is only 30%, making it difficult to resolve issues early.

• Design and implement a systematic approach/structure on how to disclose unexpected outcomes to patients and families. Effective disclosure needs to be done in a systematic and consistent fashion. Structure and ownership for the process are essential. Such a process must be created with input from multiple disciplines, including administrative leaders, medical staff leaders, attorneys, patient safety professionals, and risk managers. The process benefits from involvement of a situation management team—described below—and an individual who can mediate conversations and act as an ombudsman between the patient/family, involved practitioners, and administration. One such ombudsman/mediator role is described beginning on page 87.

• Provide regular education for providers about the importance of effective communication and how to partner with patients to achieve safe care. Effective communication begins the moment a patient enters a health care facility and meets his or her physicians. By taking the time to explain options, listen to concerns, communicate with sincerity, be humble about their abilities, and realistic about the risks and uncertainties inherent in health care, providers set the tone for collaboration and trust. If the patient perceives a provider as helpful, communicative, and honest, he or she will have more understanding in a situation in which things get out of control. Conversely, if a patient perceives a provider as removed, aloof, short-tempered, and condescending, he or she is more likely to blame the provider when a situation ends poorly. Poor relationships with physicians translate directly to lawsuits. Patients who perceive the patient-provider relationship as respectful often refuse to sue the provider; however, if the patient believes the relationship is not respectful, there can be a strong desire to name the provider in the lawsuit whether he or she is culpable or not.

The central conclusion of a study by Hickson et al. is that the inability to establish rapport with the patient is a root cause of increased risk for malpractice suits. This research shows that 6% of physicians attract 40% of lawsuits and generate 85% of malpractice losses.[18] In a study by Ambady et al., the tone of the surgeon's voice alone was linked to future malpractice claims. Four 10-second segments of the surgeon's voice were recorded at the beginning and end of patient meetings. The recordings were scrambled so that the researchers could hear only the surgeon's tone of voice. On the basis of listening to the tone of the surgeon's voice for 40 seconds, college students could predict 85% of the time the malpractice history of the physician.[19]

To achieve significant change in a provider's communication style, didactic lectures are not sufficient. When educating providers on improving communication, it is very helpful to use real scenarios in which providers can be debriefed for personal improvement. As previously mentioned, this not only provides procedural learning—"I have done this and know how"—but also helps people become more comfortable with inherently difficult conversations. From a strategic perspective, it may be useful to have the goals of broadly enhancing communication between caregivers and patients related to plans, risks, day-to-day outcomes, and informed consent. In addition, having "just in time" training and support related to disclosing major adverse events is essential.

OTHER ITEMS TO CONSIDER

Coordinating the development of a disclosure policy and accompanying procedures with your malpractice insurance company is essential to ensure that there are no conflicting messages. Hospital leaders should engage with the malpractice carrier to share their goals and discuss how the carrier can support the hospital and providers. This is particularly helpful if the hospital and providers are insured by different carriers. These discussions are helpful in supporting a rapid resolution of a case.

Organizations must make sure of the following:

• Procedures are in place and are known to bring a case to closure respectfully, as viewed by the patient and family.

• Mechanisms are in place to ensure learning by the board, executive leadership, the Medical Staff Executive Committee, and across the organization.

• Measurement systems are in place to assess the impact of communication, disclosure, and support (as well as quality and safety) practices on premiums, and to the extent possible on claims, cases, and payments.

HOW TO DISCLOSE
Disclosure Policy

As a first step, organizations need leadership commitment that open, honest disclosure is a basic component of the organizational culture. Policies should be developed that support and inform situations in which disclosure is needed. Policies should be created with input from a multidisciplinary group, including physicians, nurses, risk managers, patient safety officers, and senior leadership. Consideration should be given to involving patient representatives in policy making as well. For example, many patients who have been harmed want to hear directly from the physician involved in their care who is closest to the adverse outcome.[20]

A disclosure policy should include the following elements:

- Objectives and principles of the disclosure process. This could include the need to be honest, compassionate, and understanding in communications with patients.
- A description of the type of events that will trigger the plan
- Roles and responsibilities of health care staff and organization leadership
- Reporting process and timelines
- Checklists to help with event management
- Development of the situation management team (described below)
- A description of how compensation, outside of the payment of a malpractice claim, will be budgeted, authorized, and processed

Some other things to keep in mind when developing a policy is that when things go wrong, there are three things that patients most want:

- An honest explanation as to what happened
- An empathetic statement and apology related to the unanticipated outcome, demonstrating that the organization cares what happened to their loved one
- Information about what the organization is doing and will do to fix the problem so it won't happen to anyone else

Patients are becoming increasingly interested in wanting to be part of the solution. Maine Medical Center is now offering patients and/or families the opportunity to speak to staff and physicians, and it is videotaping their stories as a teaching tool. Another option is to embed patients onto frontline improvement teams. Of course, compensation, where warranted, may not only be an expectation, it's often the right thing to do. More information about compensation can be found on page 87.

Situation Management Team

Even with an established process for disclosure, every adverse event is different, and the specifics of the process will vary depending on what happened, the players involved, and the nature of the outcomes. To help navigate the disclosure process, organizations may want to create a situation management team (SMT). This is a multidisciplinary group that comes together to best address the nuances involved in a particular case and provide direction and support to the individuals directly working with the patients and families. Depending on the specific organization, the individuals that make up this team will vary, however core team members could include the following:

- Risk manager
- Hospital leadership
- Physician leader
- Nursing leader
- Ethicist
- Chaplain
- Individual accountable for acting as an ombudsman and/or mediator. (Note: some organizations keep this role somewhat separate from the SMT process to help preserve "neutrality" in dealings with the patient, family, and caregivers).

In specific situations, it may be helpful to include others on the SMT, such as the department head of the area in which the event occurred, the provider, a representative from public relations, or others involved in the event.[1]

Disclosure Checklist

Within the disclosure policy, organizations may also want to outline a step-by-step process that providers can use to ensure appropriate and timely disclosure. Although there are no hard-and-fast rules on how to effectively disclose information and solicit ideas or requests from patients to aid in the resolution of their event, following is one effective approach. When a major unanticipated event occurs do the following:

Immediately following patient harm:

1. Stabilize the patient.
2. Treat any injury.
3. Prevent further harm.
4. Eliminate any obvious remaining threat to patient safety, such as an impaired provider, faulty equipment, an unsafe system of care, or a seriously deficient protocol.

5. Immediately secure implicated drugs, equipment, and records.

6. Document all actions in the medical record.

7. If the primary provider is impaired, immediately provide a substitute and inform the patient and family.

8. Ensure that all members of the care team are fully aware of the issues so that subsequent communication with the patient and family is consistent.

Planning for and communicating with patients and families:

1. Engage risk management professionals.

2. Establish who will have primary responsibility for communicating with the patient and family about the event. This may be the physician or provider involved in the event, an ombudsman (often termed a *mediator*), a member of the situation management team, the risk manager, or the patient safety officer. Being in tune with what the patient/family needs and wants will serve the organization well in this area.

3. Communicate—in simple language and not medical jargon[21]—with the patient and family about the event. As soon as possible, the patient and family should learn of the event and the facts as known. Delay for the purpose of a more thorough disclosure is typically counterproductive, particularly if it is apparent that something is wrong. All communication regarding an event should involve the following:

   a. An objective description of the event

   b. Its consequences

   c. The processes being used to analyze and review systems to minimize the chances of the event recurring

   d. Ample opportunity for questions from the family.

During the disclosure, staff should refrain from offering subjective information, speculation, or beliefs relating to possible causes of the adverse event, as that can further confuse the situation and lead to possible liability. It is absolutely acceptable to say, "Here is what we know right now; there are some things we need to look at more closely and learn about; and when we have done this, we will come back and tell you." Staff must absolutely refrain from offering comments or criticisms of the health care team.

Although every effort should be made to help the patient and family, staff should not promise what cannot be delivered. This will only lead to frustration and anger on the part of the patient and family.

4. Let the patient and family know what future communication they can expect and make it clear there will be many conversations and that they will continue until the patient and family are satisfied.

5. Provide access to emotional and psychological support for the patient and family as long as it is required.

After the initial disclosure conversation:

1. Support affected members of the patient care team, sometimes referred to as the *second victims*.[3] A fundamental element involved in disclosure is leadership support for practitioners and spokespersons. Providers should not be made to feel guilty as a result of an unanticipated adverse event but, on the contrary, should feel strongly supported and valued. Physicians and other health care personnel will generally need some form of emotional support in the aftermath of a major untoward event, particularly if it involved an error. In the disclosure policy, organizations should identify individuals or departments that can provide this type of support. Scott et al. describe a rapid response system, developed and implemented at University of Missouri Health Care (Columbia), that was designed to provide social, psychological, emotional, and professional support for health care providers traumatized as a result of their involvement in an unanticipated adverse event, medical error, or patient-related injury.[22] The system entails an interprofessional *forYOU Team*—physicians, nurses, social workers, respiratory therapists, and other allied health team members who provide interventional support. A second victim support toolkit that was launched in 2010 consists of 10 modules, each with a series of specific action steps, references, and exemplars.[23,24]

2. Regarding the event itself, staff members should be provided as much information as possible and told what they can discuss and with whom. Any promises made to staff should be fulfilled.

3. Determine the circumstances surrounding the event and the contributing factors as quickly as possible while memories of those involved are fresh.

4. Report the error that resulted in an adverse event to the appropriate parties. Depending on the error, different departments, entities, or agencies may need to be notified. For example, the risk manager, patient safety officer, or quality improvement department may need to be notified.

5. As soon as practical, all involved parties should participate in a systematic analysis of the event. Generally, root cause analyses are reserved for sentinel events—a sentinel

event being "an unexpected occurrence involving death or serious physical or psychological injury, or the risk thereof"—but classified as such by the organization, which can also chose to conduct them on adverse events in general or even close calls.[6]

6. Although adverse events are difficult and painful for all involved, they do present a unique opportunity for learning. As previously discussed, organizations should carefully review the circumstances behind events and look for underlying system failures that can be addressed in order to prevent further error.

7. In follow-up meetings with the family and patient, appropriate staff should communicate the results of the analysis and corrective action plans.

8. In some cases, it may be appropriate to offer compensation, defined as "a financial remedy accorded to an individual who has sustained an arguably avoidable loss in order to replace the loss caused by the arguably inappropriate act, with the intention of making the injured party whole."[25(p. 22)] Richard Boothman (University of Michigan) notes, "Not every patient wants compensation and not all compensation is financial, but the inability or unwillingness to offer it signals insincerity and suggests that apologies are really affectations or strategies, not an integrated step borne of a commitment to honesty."[25(p. 22)]

Who Should Disclose?

Organizations have different experiences and opinions regarding what's right for them with regard to this question. Ultimately, their decision should be informed by what's right for the patient and family. It is certainly difficult to give bad news. It is even more difficult when the bad news may be the result of errors in the care delivered. Disclosure is a trained skill, and one that does not come naturally to most people. Ideally, all health care training should include effective communication and disclosure skills. In organizations delivering care, however, actually training everyone is a huge task. In addition, a provider who has been a part of an incident may not be in a position to effectively communicate with the patient and family, and an impartial perspective may be beneficial. However, if the patient and family have a trusting relationship with the provider, he or she should be able to gain their understanding.

To address these issues, one approach to consider is training a few individuals to become "experts" in disclosure.

These individuals come on site when there is a disclosure situation to aid the physician and facilitate direct communication with staff, the patient, and his or her family. These individuals should be trained and given the tools to have effective conversations. They should be compassionate individuals with excellent communication skills who are able to look at a situation from multiple vantage points.

An alternative approach is to provide some basic "communicating unanticipated adverse outcomes" training to physicians, and support them with both a situation management team for appropriate response strategies shortly after the event, and a skilled ombudsman for assistance in longer-term conversations with the patient or family. As stated earlier, most patients want to hear from their physician and/or the involved physician(s), and not a third party with whom they have no relationship.[20]

THE BENEFITS OF A HEALTH CARE OMBUDSMAN/MEDIATOR (HCOM) PROGRAM

A health care ombudsman/mediator (HCOM) program offers an opportunity for an institution to address patient and organizational concerns in a fair and just manner. This type of program is not designed to minimize malpractice. An ombudsman participates in disclosure conversations with patients and families, works to resolve issues and answer questions associated with an event, and acts as a go-between for the organization and the patient and family. An ombudsman functions independently of the organization and reports directly to the CEO or other senior leader. Neither an advocate for the patient nor for the institution, the ombudsman is an advocate for a fair process. He or she interviews all participants in an event to try to get answers for the patient. He or she also works with the patient and family to determine their needs regarding the situation. Confidentiality is maintained, and information shared in confidence with the ombudsman is not disclosed, similar to the confidentiality required of a mediator.

The following hypothetical example shows one way an ombudsman program can be used:

During Mr. White's hand surgery, the surgeon operates on the wrong hand. As soon as the surgeon realizes the error, he contacts the ombudsman, who comes to the operating room. After the patient is stabilized, the surgeon talks to the ombudsman about what happened. The ombudsman then convenes the situation management team.

The situation management team talks about the event and determines what is known, what can be shared immediately with the patient and family, what needs to be further investigated, who should communicate with the patient and family, and who will do the investigation. The group also discusses the best methods for communicating with the patient and family.

When the situation management team meets, the ombudsman and the surgeon meet with the family. The surgeon and ombudsman take the family to a private location to discuss the situation. They engage in a compassionate and honest conversation with the family, explaining what happened, what is occurring right now, and what is still not known. During the conversation, both the ombudsman and the surgeon are careful to communicate the facts that are known at the time, rather than conjecture, and make sure their explanations are understandable and empathetic.

They also discuss how they are going to continue to care for the patient and what he should expect. In this case, the surgeon offers to continue providing care—the patient still needs the intended surgery—and also offers the option of another surgeon taking over the care if that is the patient's preference. There is also a conversation about what steps will be taken to rectify the situation, as in a waiver of fees or other appropriate measures.

After the initial conversation takes place, the surgeon returns to his work while the ombudsman remains with the family to further answer any questions and identify any logistical needs the family might have. The ombudsman works to meet the immediate needs of the family and identifies any additional information that is necessary.

When the family understands the situation, the ombudsman leaves the family and updates the situation management team. The ombudsman remains in close contact with the family, following up regularly to ensure that they have no further questions. Often, the first meeting is pretty shocking, and the family doesn't have time to develop questions. Sometimes they don't even hear everything that is said. That is why it is important to contact them later to follow up on questions and ensure that they are aware of what is going on.

After the initial disclosure conversation, the organization works to investigate the event. As a result of this investigation, the organization puts protocols in place and educates the staff on these protocols to prevent such an event from happening again. The surgeon and ombudsman meet with the patient and family, take responsibility for the event, and offer an apology. They show the patient the protocols that have been put in place and also share information about the education provided to the staff on preventing wrong-site surgeries.

While Mr. White is frustrated about the operation, he appreciates the organization's candor and apology and is pleased it has implemented systems to prevent the event from happening to someone else. Mr. White and his family express gratitude for the organization's honesty and compassion. Mr. White and the surgeon shake hands.

Who Makes a Good Ombudsman

The ideal ombudsman has strong interpersonal skills, understands medical terminology and medical records, knows the organizational structure of the organization, and is respected by the providers who ultimately must place their trust in him or her. The key skill necessary for an effective ombudsman is communication. The ombudsman relies heavily on shuttle diplomacy, problem solving, and interpersonal communication skills. He or she should receive significant training in mediation and ombudsman skills, participate in one-on-one coaching for a period of time while establishing his or her position within the health care setting, and participate in regularly scheduled reflective practice and advanced trainings to further develop his or her conflict resolution and communication skills. Kaiser Permanente has extensive experience with this concept, having implemented its HCOM program in more than 30 hospitals. The authors are happy to share information about the collective experience.

CONCLUSION

Effective disclosure is very difficult and takes great skill. Being involved in a situation in which a patient has experienced avoidable harm pushes every button clinicians have with regard to whether they are competent, were paying enough attention, and were trying hard enough. Such situations are often seriously threatening to their sense of self-esteem, as they have all been taught repeatedly that "good doctors and nurses don't make mistakes," and now they are dealing with one on a profound level.

When we deal with patients and their families in these very difficult and delicate situations, we need to do something that feels vulnerable and threatening—openly engage the patient and his or her family, even if they are angry and frustrated. All too often, we back off, and the patient perceives neglect and abandonment in the setting in which he or she was harmed.

Effective disclosure requires structure, skill, and organizational commitment. The benefit is that it offers great value to patients and families as well as clinicians and the organization as a whole.

REFERENCES

1. Leonard M, Frankel A, Simmonds T, editors: *Achieving Safe and Reliable Healthcare: Strategies and Solutions.* Chicago: Health Administration Press, 2004.

2. Massachusetts Coalition for the Prevention of Medical Errors. *When Things Go Wrong: Responding to Adverse Events. A Consensus Statement of the Harvard Hospitals.* Mar 2006. Accessed Oct 31, 2012. http://www.macoalition.org/documents/respondingToAdverseEvents.pdf.

3. Wu AW. Medical error: The second victim. *BMJ.* 2000 Mar 18;320(7237):726–727.

4. Kachalia A, et al. Liability claims and costs before and after implementation of a medical error disclosure program. *Ann Intern Med.* 2010 Aug 17;153(4):213–221.

5. Agency for Healthcare Research and Quality. Medical Liability Reform and Patient Safety Initiative. Feb 2012. Accessed Oct 31, 2012. http://www.ahrq.gov/qual/liability/.

6. The Joint Commission: *2012 Comprehensive Accreditation Manual for Hospitals: The Official Handbook.* Oak Brook, IL: Joint Commission Resources, 2011.

7. National Quality Forum (NQF). *Safe Practices for Better Healthcare— 2006 Update: A Consensus Report.* Washington, DC: NQF, 2006..

8. American Medical Association (AMA). Patient information. In *Code of Medical Ethics of the American Medical Association: Current Opinions with Annotations, 2010–2011 ed.* Chicago: AMA, 2010. Accessed Oct 31, 2012. http://www.ama-assn.org/ama/pub/physician-resources/medical-ethics/code-medical-ethics.page.

9. Australian Council for Safety and Quality in Health Care. *Open Disclosure Standard: A National Standard for Open Communication in Public and Private Hospitals Following an Adverse Event in Health Care.* Canberra, Australia: Commonwealth of Australia, 2003. Accessed Oct 31, 2012. http://www.safetyandquality.health.wa.gov.au/docs/open_disclosure/ACSQHC_Open_Disclosure_Standard.pdf.

10. Canadian Patient Safety Institute. *Canadian Disclosure Guidelines: Being Open with Patients and Families.* Ottawa: Canadian Patient Safety Institute, 2011. Accessed Oct 31, 2012. http://www.patientsafetyinstitute.ca/English/toolsResources/disclosure/Pages/default.aspx.

11. NHS Lanarkshire. *Being Open: Communicating Patient Safety Incidents with Patients and Their Carers.* Mar 29, 2010. Kirklands, UK: NHS Lanarkshire. Accessed Oct 31, 2012. http://www.nhslanarkshire.org.uk/publications/Documents/Being%20Open.pdf.

12. Stokes SL, Wu AW, Pronovost PJ. Ethical and practical aspects of disclosing adverse events in the emergency department. *Emerg Med Clin North Am.* 2006;24(3):703–714.

13. Loren DJ, et al. Risk managers, physicians, and disclosure of harmful medical errors. *Jt Comm J Qual Patient Saf.* 2010;36(3):101–108.

14. Iedema R, et al. What prevents incident disclosure, and what can be done to promote it? *Jt Comm J Qual Patient Saf.* 2011;37(9):409–417.

15. Hickson GB, et al. Factors that prompted families to file medical malpractice claims following perinatal injuries. *JAMA.* 1992 Mar 11;267(10):1359–1363.

16. Wu AW: Handling hospital errors: Is disclosure the best defense? *Ann Intern Med.* 1999 Dec 21;131(12):970–972.

17. Kraman SS, Hamm G. Risk management: Extreme honesty may be the best policy. *Ann Intern Med.* 1999 Dec 21;131(12):963–967.

18. Hickson GB, et al. Patient complaints and malpractice risk. *JAMA.* 2002 Jun 12;287(22):2951–2957.

19. Ambady N, et al. Surgeons' tone of voice: A clue to malpractice history. *Surgery.* 2002;132(1):5–9,

20. Iedema RA, et al. The National Open Disclosure Pilot: Evaluation of a policy implementation initiative. *Med J Aust.* 2008 Apr 7;188(7):397-400.

21. Peto RR, et al. One system's journey in creating a disclosure and apology program. *Jt Comm J Qual Patient Saf.* 2009;35(10):487-496.

22. Scott SD, et al. Caring for our own: Deploying a systemwide second victim rapid response team. *Jt Comm J Qual Patient Saf.* 2010;36(5):233–240.

23. Pratt S, et al. How to develop a second victim support program: A toolkit for health care organizations. *Jt Comm J Qual Patient Saf.* 2012;38(5):235-240.

24. MITSS (Medically Induced Trauma Support Services). MITSS Tools: Tools for Building a Clinician and Staff Support Program. 2010. Accessed Oct 31, 2012. http://www.mitsstools.org/tool-kit-for-staff-support-for-healthcare-organizations.html.

25. Conway J, et al. *Respectful Management of Serious Clinical Adverse Events,* 2nd ed. IHI Innovation Series white paper. Cambridge, MA: Institute for Healthcare Improvement, 2011. Accessed Oct 31, 2012. http://www.ihi.org/knowledge/Pages/IHIWhitePapers/RespectfulManagementSeriousClinicalAEsWhitePaper.aspx.

Chapter Nine

ENSURING PATIENT INVOLVEMENT AND FAMILY ENGAGEMENT

*Mary Ann Abrams, MD, MPH; Gail Nielsen, BSHCA, FAHRA, RTR;
Karen Frush, BSN, MD; Barbara Balik, RN, EdD*

As discussed in Chapter 6, teamwork is a critical component in providing safe and reliable care. Essential members of the team often overlooked are the patient and family. Organizations with a reliable and safe culture design and deliver care in partnership with the patient and family, engage patients to participate in their care at the level they choose, and actively work to include patient perspectives in improvement. Such organizations partner with patients, gather feedback about their care experiences, and actively seek to understand the type of care they want.

The Internet, social and mainstream media, and increased consumerism, among many other factors, have led to an increasingly well-informed patient who has specific expectations for his or her health care experience. At the same time, millions of adults in the United States struggle with literacy and, for various reasons, have not mastered technologic innovations that can foster knowledge acquisition. Nevertheless, patients are often very aware when care doesn't go well and can provide unique insight into an organization's processes and procedures.[1] Health care organizations cannot afford to ignore this essential resource.

Organizations that create opportunities for patients and their families (patients/families), and staff to work together can accelerate improvement in the safety and quality of the care experience. The Joint Commission's "Provision of Care" (PC) chapter includes Standard PC.02.03.01, "The hospital provides patient education and training based on each patient's needs and abilities"; Element of Performance (EP) 1 ("The hospital performs a learning needs assessment for each patient, which includes the patient's cultural and religious beliefs, emotional barriers, desire and motivation to learn, physical or cognitive limitations, and barriers to communication"); and EP 27 ("The hospital provides the patient education on how to communicate concerns about patient safety issues that occur before, during, and after care is received.")[2] In addition, the Rights and Responsibilities Standard RI.01.01.01 states, "The hospital respects, protects, and promotes patient rights"; EP 28 stipulates, "The hospital allows a family member, friend, or other individual to be present with the patient for emotional support during the course of stay." Leadership Standard LD.03.04.01 states, "The hospital communicates information related to safety and quality to those who need it, including staff, licensed independent practitioners, patients, families, and external interested parties."[2]

Engaging patients and designated family members in their care has many benefits, including the following:
- Ensures the most appropriate care for the patient
- Respects any specific cultural or emotional needs
- Improves patient outcomes[3]
- Helps identify potential system issues or gaps in care
- Helps improve staff satisfaction and provider engagement

Despite its many benefits, involving patients/families in their care conflicts with an old but still present philosophy of the clinician as the individual provider and the patient as the recipient, not participant, in his or her care. Achieving a culture centered on the patient takes bold leadership. Leadership must embrace the concept of patient/family partnership, promote it among staff and patients, and invest in resources and training to build the collaborative skills of staff and providers.

WAYS TO PARTNER WITH PATIENTS

There are many ways to partner with patients in the care delivery process. The following sections examine a few of these ways.

Partner with Patients and Caregivers in Treatment Shared Care Planning

Partnering with patients in their treatment decisions helps individuals to understand their illness and treatment options and can also help them recognize when treatment deviates from expected. This not only respects the patient's rights and preferences but can help organizations identify errors and point out inconsistencies (*see* Sidebar 9-1, right). Organizations can partner with patients in their care by taking some of the following steps:

• Shared care plans. This can be accomplished through continuous conversation among the care team, including the patient/family, with mutual goal-setting about the type of treatment a patient needs and the state of his or her recovery. These conversations occur during multidisciplinary bedside rounds, during transitions in care, and at change-of-shift report.

• Review daily goals. A daily goal sheet outlines every goal for the patient for a particular day or shift. These goals, which may address physical, emotional, or spiritual aspects of care, are areas in which the patient needs to have significant input. An example of a clinical (physical) goal would be to take the patient off his or her ventilator by the end of the day. An emotional goal might be that the patient experiences less fear while being weaned from the ventilator. Whatever the goals listed on the daily goal sheets, the clinicians should discuss and review them with the patient/family and incorporate their contributions. The daily or shift goals should be written on the whiteboard in the patient's room. This way all staff associated with the patient's care can be on the same page as to what the patient's goals are for treatment.

• Conduct multidisciplinary bedside rounds that actively involve and engage the patient/family. As discussed in Chapter 6, these are done at shift change and throughout the day so that all team members are aware of the treatment plan, daily goals, and progress toward meeting those goals.

• Involve the patient in handoffs when his or her care is handed off from one provider to another. Introducing the patient to the new provider, updating the patient on the status of achieving outcomes and goals, and reassessing the

---

Sidebar 9-1. Empowering Patients to Speak Up

In March 2002 The Joint Commission, together with the Centers for Medicare & Medicaid Services (CMS), launched a national campaign to urge patients to take a role in preventing health care errors by becoming active, involved, and informed participants on the health care team. The program features free, downloadable brochures, posters, and buttons on a variety of patient safety topics, including the following[1]:
• Preventing errors
• Avoiding mistakes in surgery
• Information for living organ donors
• Five things to prevent infection
• Avoiding mistakes with medicines
• Research studies
• Follow-up care
• Preventing medical test mistakes
• Patient rights
• Understanding physicians and other caregivers
• Pain management
• Reducing the risk of falling
• Five ways to be active in your care (diabetes, dialysis)

Within each topic, the Speak Up™ campaign encourages the public to do the following:

Speak up if you have questions or concerns, and if you don't understand, ask again. It's your body and you have a right to know.

Pay attention to the care you are receiving. Make sure you're getting the right treatments and medications by the right health care professionals. Don't assume anything.

Educate yourself about your diagnosis, the medical tests you are undergoing, and your treatment plan.

Ask a trusted family member or friend to be your advocate.

Know what medications you take and why you take them. Medication errors are the most common health care mistakes.

Use a hospital, clinic, surgery center, or other type of health care organization that has undergone a rigorous on-site evaluation against established state-of-the-art quality and safety standards, such as that provided by The Joint Commission.

Participate in all decisions about your treatment. You are the center of the health care team.

Reference
1. The Joint Commission. Speak Up Initiatives. Accessed Oct 31, 2012. http://www.jointcommission.org/speakup.aspx.

---

patient's feelings about those goals can all be helpful at this time. Kaiser Permanente uses a process called the Nurse Knowledge Exchange to involve patients in the handoff process.[4] Nurses hand off patient care at the bedside with the patients and family. Using a Situation, Background, Assessment, Recommendation (SBAR) format, called I-SBAR—I standing for Introduce—nurses communicate with the patient about the status of his or her care and what he or she can expect during the next shift. They also introduce the nurse taking over care, so the patient can associate a face with a name. Nurses have a 60-second framing conversation before going into the patient's room to help focus the conversation and determine two to three items to keep on the front burner. Some units incorporate a whiteboard in the process so the nurse can write down what's going to happen, and patients/families can document any questions for the next exchange. Nurses finish the process by asking patients to "teach-back" the material covered in the exchange. At this time they also invite patient/family questions or correct information they believe is inaccurate. (*See* pages 99–100 for more information on the teach-back method.)

• Engage the patient/family in the discharge handoff process. On admission, throughout the hospital or skilled nursing care facility stay, and in preparing for discharge, the patient/family should be part of the planning regarding the patient's needs in returning home.

• Involve patients to the extent that they desire in their care. This means that patients should be informed about any test results, treatment plans, protocols, and procedures, as well as selective education about their care that is targeted to their reading level and immediate needs rather than trying to teach all components at once. (*See* pages 96–101 for more information on patient education.) As specified by Joint Commission National Patient Safety Goal NPSG.07.03.01 ("Implement evidence-based practices to prevent health care–associated infections due to multidrug-resistant organisms in acute care hospitals"), education should address the actions—such as hand hygiene and contact precautions—that patients/families can take to help prevent health care–associated infections, including surgical site infections.[2]

Listen to and Learn from Patient and Family Feedback

As previously mentioned, the nuances of the care experience are not lost on patients. They are acutely aware of the efficiency (or lack thereof) of the care they receive, how well the providers "get along," and how well they feel when leaving the facility. In addition, patients/families may know more about thier journey across the continuum of care, across boundaries and sites of care than many providers. They know the "white spaces" between providers and organizations. They have knowledge we do not have to keep them safe in transitions. Organizations should tap into this wealth of knowledge to help identify gaps in care and areas of opportunity. Following are some sources for patient feedback:

• Patient experience surveys
• Observations of the patient/family experience of care
• Focus groups
• Compliment/complaint letters
• Safety hotlines
• Staff feedback
• Community groups
• Patient/family council advisors[1] (*see* Sidebar 9-2, pages 94–95)
• Patients as members of the patient safety and other committees

Information from these feedback sources should be analyzed and prioritized along with other issue identification and performance data. The patient safety officer plays a critical role in reviewing, analyzing, and prioritizing these data.

Partner with Patients and Their Families to Improve Care Across the Organization

To truly partner with patients/families, you must involve them at the policy-making level. This may mean inviting them to participate on your organization's quality or safety committee, sentinel event review panel, or other performance improvement–related committee. Although some organizations may balk at this idea, given their perception that it might expose them to potential lawsuits or bad press, other organizations have embraced the concept, choosing to learn from patient perspectives and experiences rather than trying to deny them. Consider this example:

A patient/family advisor whose mother contracted Clostridium difficile *while hospitalized joined the safety and quality committee. In setting improvement goals for hand hygiene for the following year, the clinicians and staff on the committee had an extended conversation about what was an achievable goal—should it be 85% or 87%? The patient/family advisor listened respectfully then asked, "Why isn't it 100%?" The nature of the conversation changed dramatically to how fast they could achieve 100%.*

Sidebar 9-2. Patient and Family Advisors and Patient and Family Councils

Patient and Family Advisors

Patient and family (P/F) advisors offer an abundance of help to transform health care. Their perspective brings focus, urgency, and clarity to improving the safety and quality of care. A way to begin this partnership is by identifying small projects the P/F advisors can participate in to build both their and the organization's skills in partnership.

Ways to begin include the following:
- Be clear on why you want P/F advisors. An example is—"Patient and/or family member partnerships and participation is essential to improved health and healing in health care organizations."
- Be clear on your purpose for partnerships with patients and families on improvement work, teams, councils, and so on. What outcomes are you seeking that those partnerships will help achieve?

P/F advisors can contribute in a variety of ways. Here are some steps to take:
- Identify where you need P/F participation
  - Offer a range of options to potential P/F advisors. Start small—avoid a Patient/Family Advisory Council as a first step. A one-to-two-session commitment or those that can be done at home by P/F advisors offers a test of the P/F advisor's capacity to contribute and the staff/leaders' ability to work effectively in partnership. This also can limit the risk for both parties if it is not a match or the staff are not ready to work in partnership.
- Activities might include the following:
  - Codevelopment of new patient education materials
  - Review of existing patient education materials
  - Review of proposed changes to an existing program
  - Design of new program
  - Design of new space
  - "Sharing their story" during staff orientation
  - Interview of candidates for key positions; for example, at one organization, cancer survivors or family members interview candidates for oncology care navigator positions.
- Given the purpose, what skills are sought from an advisor? Some examples include the following:
  - Shares insights about his or her experiences in ways that others can learn from them
  - Sees beyond his or her personal experiences to understand others' experiences
  - Shows concern for more than one issue, not focused on one agenda only
  - Listens well and respects others' perspectives; a good partner
  - Eager to contribute to improved care; wants to give back
  - "Constructively disgruntled," that is, he or she may not think that the organization is perfect (not a cheerleader) but wants it to succeed (loyal)
  - Interacts well with different kinds of people
  - Speaks comfortably in a group with candor
  - Represents the patients served, including cultural, racial, or ethnic communities

  - Stakeholders in the topic at hand
- Go with someone who will be successful—think of someone you would ask to be on the board.
- Given the skills, write a "position description" specifying the following:
  - Project purpose
  - Skills sought
  - Expectations: what you want the advisor to do
  - Meeting times, frequency, and time commitment
  - Expenses covered (for example, parking, meals, child care costs)
  - What they can expect from health care leaders to support their work as an advisor
  - Training provided
- Given the skills, identify potential members:
  - Ask clinicians, "Do you know a patient/family member who comes to mind as a potential member?"
  - Are there patients/family members who have contacted health care leaders about concerns and who were highly effective in communicating their requests?
  - Are there P/Fs with unique perspectives as previous patients or family caregivers for a project?
  - Use your internal and external network of Board members, faith community, volunteers to cast a wide search

Recruitment:
- If a potential P/F advisor is suggested by a clinician, ask the clinician to contact the P/F to invite him or her to learn more.
- Have the key contact call the P/F to set up a face-to-face meeting (at a location convenient for the P/F, such as a coffee shop) to review the following:
  - Information on the options to participate
  - Position description
- Reconnect in one week to address questions and agree on participation.

Orientation:
- Use current volunteer screening and orientation
  - Include confidentiality statement that meets requirements for HIPAA* compliance.

Organization overview
- Project specifics, including aim and time frame
- Where this project fits in the organization's mission
- Meeting facilitation and ground rules
  - Ice breakers
  - Participation
  - What to do when you disagree
  - Active listening
  - Speaking up when staff use language you do not understand

---

* US Department of Health & Human Services. HIPAA Administrative Simplification Statute and Rules. Accessed Oct 31, 2012. http://www.hhs.gov/ocr/privacy/hipaa/administrative/index.html.

Sidebar 9-2. Patient and Family Advisors and Patient and Family Councils (continued)

Patient and Family Council

One specific way to engage patients is to create a patient and family council.[1] These councils, typically made up of mostly patients and supported by health care system representatives from operations, administration, and quality, help ensure that the patient experience, point of view, and recommendations are shared in a way that creates greater respect for and profound knowledge concerning the fundamental question: "What is in the best interest of the patient?" The council can meet regularly to provide input on patient care, review patient satisfaction survey results, serve as a resource for improvement initiatives throughout the organization, and initiate its own improvement projects. For example, if your department was working on a fall prevention initiative, you could solicit the patient and family council and ask for help with that project. The council could identify a liaison who would work directly with your performance improvement team.

A patient and family council can show firsthand your organization's commitment to patient involvement in care and provide a venue for patients and families to give valuable feedback in real time. Patients provide a unique perspective and, when designing any new program or process, having them involved helps ensure that the process is as good as it can be. For example, before launching an initiative, your organization can test the concept with the patient and family council and receive honest, real-time feedback about the concept without having to wait three to four months for patient satisfaction survey results.

One organization that is very familiar with the concept of a patient and family council is the Dana-Farber Cancer

Institute. The hospital's patient and family council has accomplished much in its 10-year existence. For instance, the group produces a newsletter written for patients and families by patients and families; participates in legislative activity; and helps teach other organizations how to implement patient/family-centered programs.

The hospital supplies a small budget, but all decisions in the council are made independently by council members. Recently, Dana-Farber began designing and building a new oncology and ambulatory care center. Council members were involved in the planning and helped choose the architect. Council members also participate in developing staff education materials. For example, council members were involved in creating a video on informed consent in which they gave input on how physicians can encourage patients to enroll in clinical trials and also respect patients who are not interested in being a part of clinical trials. The council also helped establish a fast-track process for children with a fever and low white blood cell count in the emergency department.

The role of the patient and family council is valued at all levels of Dana-Farber. An individual cannot be hired into a senior-level position without being interviewed by a member of the patient council.

Reference

1. Dana-Farber Cancer Institute. Establishing Patient- and Family-Centered Care. Accessed Oct 31, 2012. http://www.danafarber.org/Adult-Care/New-Patient-Guide/Adult-Patient-and-Family-Advisory-Council/Establishing-Patient-and-Family-Centered-Care.aspx.

Patients/families should also be directly involved in the design and improvement of programs that affect patients. For example, if your organization is creating a new website, involve patients/families in that process. They can provide unique feedback on the site's ease of use and the appropriateness of the content and flow.

Similarly, patients/families can be assets in improving wayfinding in health care settings, which may improve access and the likelihood of follow-through on appointments. Walk with patients as they navigate their way to specific locations for appointments and testing; learn from them and provide this information to other patients.[5]

Involve Patients in Provider Education

There is no better way to educate physicians, nurses, and other direct care providers on the importance of communicating effectively with patients than to have a patient share

his or her care experiences with the team. Providers may not be aware of how their tone, mannerisms, and bedside manner affect patients, but listening to a patient share his or her care experience can sometimes bring new insight to clinicians. Patient/family advisors can be highly effective in assisting with orientation of new staff and providers through sharing their stories and describing what matters to them most.

Some institutions are including patients and patient advocates as instructors in training courses for clinicians. Duke University Health System (DUHS) is one of seven national training sites for the TeamSTEPPS® National Implementation program.[6] TeamSTEPPS is an evidence-based, train-the-trainer curriculum that teaches effective communication and teamwork skills to participants through didactic lectures and small-group interactive sessions. At DUHS, leaders have invited members of its

Patient Advocacy Council (composed of volunteer patients and community members), to be trained as TeamSTEPPS Master Trainers along with clinicians. As Master Trainers, patient advocates can then participate on instructor-teams with clinician trainers, and teach future TeamSTEPPS courses. Patient safety leaders at DUHS believe that these clinician/patient instructor teams provide a model of the institution's commitment to facilitating patient engagement and strengthening the provider/patient partnership.

Involve the Family Whenever Possible

Undergoing medical procedures can be intimidating, but being separated from loved ones who can provide support makes even routine procedures more stressful. Organizations that include families in the care of patients have observed improved clinical outcomes, as well as increased patient satisfaction with the quality of care.[7,8]

Families should be part of any education provided to patients, and they should be encouraged to participate in treatment decisions when appropriate. One way to encourage family involvement is to ensure family presence by maintaining open access to nursing units, ICUs, and the emergency department. By keeping these areas open to families 24 hours a day—even during shift changes, rounds, resuscitation events, and other emergency situations—you can encourage their involvement, decrease the potential for error, and increase patient safety. Similarly, those organizations that allow family members to stay during anesthesia induction, in the recovery room, in radiology, and during treatment and procedures open up the environment and reduce the potential for errors.[8]

ADDRESSING PATIENT LITERACY

Ninety million adults in the United States read below high school level. People with limited reading skills are less likely to use preventive health measures; less likely to know about their illnesses, their medicines, and how to care for themselves; more likely to be hospitalized; and more likely to die earlier.[9,10] Clearly, health literacy is fundamental to safe, high-quality care.[9]

Health literacy is defined by the Institute of Medicine as "the degree to which individuals have the capacity to obtain, process, and understand basic health information and services needed to make appropriate health decisions."[9(p. 32),11]

The 2003 National Assessment of Adult Literacy showed that 88% of adults in the United States lack proficient health literacy, impeding their ability to use the health care system.[12] People with low health literacy can have problems with medications, over-the-counter drug dose calculations, appointment slips, consent forms, discharge instructions, health education materials and insurance applications. They have trouble understanding this information, following treatment plans, and seeking follow-up care, and may be unwilling or unable to ask questions.

Consider this example: Mr. Jones is a diabetic patient who recently was given instructions on how to take his insulin. Unbeknownst to his nurse, Mr. Jones cannot read. Although Mr. Jones is conscientious about taking his medicine and eating the proper foods, he is admitted to the ICU three times over three months for severe diabetic ketoacidosis, a potentially life-threatening condition. During his third admission to the ICU, the nurse, sensing something is wrong, meets with Mr. Jones and asks him to describe his diet and show how he gives himself insulin shots. Mr. Jones says that he is not able to show the nurse because he does not have an orange, and frankly, he's getting a little tired of oranges and is there any other way to administer the medication. The nurse realizes that the patient had been taught to administer insulin by injecting it into oranges, and he went home and continued to do so, eating the oranges, rather than injecting the insulin into himself! Three trips to the ICU and roughly $100,000 of cost occurred because the organization didn't effectively teach the patient how to correctly administer his insulin. Mr. Jones didn't know, and the people providing care had no idea.

Low health literacy is associated with more hospitalizations; greater use of emergency care; lower receipt of mammography screening and influenza vaccine; poorer ability to demonstrate taking medications appropriately; poorer ability to interpret labels and health messages; and, among elderly persons, poorer health status and higher mortality outcomes.[10]

How Do You Know If a Patient Has a Literacy Problem?

Low literacy is not necessarily obvious, and a patient can look and speak in a way that does not suggest a problem with health literacy. Anyone—regardless of age, race, education, or income—can have problems with health literacy. Older patients, recent immigrants, and people with chronic disease are especially vulnerable to low health literacy. People who can't read or understand health care information are often ashamed of this and are very good at hiding the problem. According to one study, 70% of people who cannot read do not tell their spouse.[13] If they aren't going to tell their loved ones they can't read, what makes us think they will tell us?

Although it is hard to tell when someone is struggling with reading, there are potential signs[14]:

- It takes the patient longer to fill out a form.
- The patient "forgets" to bring his or her glasses and asks the provider to read the form aloud or asks for permission to take it home to fill it out.
- The patient never asks questions. This may be a personality trait or cultural barrier, but it could also be an indication that the patient does not understand the information provided.
- You observe the patient struggling to read.
- The patient asks "where do I sign?" versus "do I sign here?"
- The patient continuously misses appointments. If your organization communicates information about the next appointment using a written appointment card, and the patient cannot read, he or she will rely on memory to keep the appointment, and as we already know, human memory is fallible.

Patients with low literacy may bring someone who can read with them to their appointment, watch other people and do what they do, pretend they can read, or ask for help from other patients or staff. Most patients with low literacy, however, never ask for help.[13]

Why Address Patient Literacy?

Low health literacy is not only dangerous for the patient; it costs the health care system in the United States an estimated $106–$236 billion a year.[15] Treatments for congestive heart failure, asthma, and diabetes make up a large portion of health care spending, and many of the individuals receiving those treatments have low health literacy. If health care organizations designed services to address low health literacy among patients with those chronic conditions, the health care system could reduce the cost of health care. A safer health care environment is one in which patients understand what is happening to them, make *informed* health decisions, know what their role is in their care, and do not experience

a sense of shame or embarrassment at any time.[16] A critical way to achieve this environment is to ensure that education provided to patients is simple, straightforward, understandable, and sensitive to cultural needs.

In 2010 three major US government initiatives—the Affordable Care Act, the Department of Health and Human Services' National Action Plan to Improve Health Literacy, and the Plain Writing Act of 2010—addressed health literacy and prioritized it as an access, quality, and cost issue for public and private health care organizations.[17] If public and private organizations make it a priority to become health literate, health literacy could be advanced to the point at which it would play a major role in improving health care and health for all Americans.[17]

Make It Simple for Everyone

Some organizations believe in assessing general reading levels to help determine health literacy; however, assessing literacy levels does not ensure patient understanding in the clinical setting.[16] The best approach to educating patients is to worry less about identifying people who struggle with literacy and instead recognize that low health literacy is a universal problem. If you spend a lot of time trying to separate the literate from those who struggle to read, you may overlook the fact that when stressed, worried, or ill, even the most literate individuals may fail to understand and remember complex information. All patients appreciate simple, easy-to-understand information focused on what they need to know. Highly literate individuals are not offended by simple, clear communication.

Like so many aspects of the health care delivery process, to truly address low health literacy in health care organizations, you must take a systematic approach. This requires leadership support, effective tools, and comprehensive training for providers on how to educate patients and overcome literacy issues. Following are some tips that organizations can use to help develop a systematic approach:

- Include the need to address health literacy in the strategic plan. This helps ensure continual resources dedicated to patient education and health literacy.
- Foster an environment in which providers communicate openly and respectfully with patients, encouraging them to speak up and be involved in their care.
- Provide a shame-free environment in which patients feel comfortable saying that they don't understand, asking

---

Sidebar 9-3. Informed Consent

Low health literacy can be an important issue in the informed consent process. A 2009 systematic review showed the majority of studies on informed consent for surgery show inadequate to moderate understanding of information provided to patients, including risks and benefits of the procedure.[1] This creates a significant patient safety issue.

To prevent possible harm or risk associated with a patient's lack of understanding, organizations should review their informed consent processes and ensure that the forms used to document the informed consent discussion between providers and patients are written in an appropriate, easy-to-understand manner. If they are not, revising the forms using plain language principles should be considered (see pages 97–98).

To support overarching health literacy goals of improving interpersonal and written communication and creating a patient-centered care environment through use of plain language principles and the teach-back method, in 2004 Iowa Health System enhanced its process for obtaining and documenting informed consent for surgery from patients to promote patient understanding. A health literacy–based, reader-friendly consent for surgery/procedures that included space to record patients' description of their procedure in their own words was developed in collaboration with health literacy teams, adult learners, risk managers, health care providers, and the law department. Comparison between surgical patients at hospitals that did and did not use the revised form showed that patients in hospitals using the form were more likely to recall being asked to describe their surgery in their own words and reported enhanced comfort with asking questions about their surgery.

A health literacy–based reader-friendly consent can drive use of teach-back and enhance safety by promoting clear communication in this important setting.[2]

It may be helpful to test new or revised documents with a sample of patients from diverse backgrounds. Questions to ask could include the following:
• Given the time, were you able to finish reading the form?

• Can you describe what the form says? How easy is it for you to do that?
• Do you have any questions about the form? Was anything unclear?
• Were there any words on the form you did not understand?

Consider the following example: The first paragraph is an organization's original consent form. The second paragraph is the revision using shorter sentences and plain language.

Old
It has been explained to me that during the course of the operation, unforeseen conditions may be revealed that necessitate an extension of the original procedure(s) or different procedure(s) than those described above. I, therefore, authorize such surgical procedure(s) as are necessary and desirable in the exercise of the professional judgment. The authority granted under this shall extend to all conditions that do require treatment even if not known to Dr. _____ at the time the operation is commenced.

New
I understand the doctor may find other medical conditions he/she did not expect during my surgery or procedure. I agree that my doctor may do any extra treatments or procedures he/she thinks are needed for medical reasons during my surgery or procedure.

It is key that in addition to improving the consent form, your organization reviews the processes around informed consent. Providers should use easy-to-understand language when explaining the procedure and use the teach-back method to confirm understanding.

References
1. Falagas ME, et al. Informed consent: How much and what do patients understand? *Am J Surg.* 2009;198(3):420–435.
2. Miller MJ, et al. Improving patient-provider communication for patients having surgery: Patient perceptions of a revised health literacy-based consent process. *J Patient Saf.* 2011;7(1):30–38.

Source: Gail Nielsen, Iowa Health System. Used with permission.

---

questions, and talking openly about their health and concerns. Organizations can achieve such an environment by encouraging staff to have an attitude of helpfulness, caring, and respect; providing easy-to-follow instructions for appointments, check-in, referrals, and tests; having simple telephone processes; providing confidential assistance; and ensuring that all staff members understand their role in enhancing patient understanding.[14]

• Reinforce the universal nature of the problem of understanding in the complex healthcare environment. The US Agency for Healthcare Research and Quality Health Literacy Universal Precautions Toolkit offers primary care practices a way to assess their services for health literacy considerations, raise awareness of the entire staff, and work on specific areas.[18] It can also be adapted for use in hospitals and other patient care settings.

• Create patient-friendly education materials (*see* Sidebar 9-3, above). Written education, when done well, can be a helpful supplement to the patient-provider conversation. Often, however, such materials include complex medical terms, are written at a level above the patient's ability to understand, contain too much information, and are not designed to be easy to read. To help improve the likelihood that written materials will be effective, consider the following strategies (*see* Sidebar 9-4, at right):

—Use simple words (1–2 syllables), short sentences (4–6 words), and short paragraphs (2–3 sentences).

—Separate text with headings and bullets.

—Incorporate lots of white space.

—Avoid medical jargon.

—Prominently locate the vital "need-to-know" information.

—Use drawings and pictures to illustrate points. These should support the text; be simple, realistic, and culturally appropriate; and show the correct way to do things.

—Make the font size easy to read—14 point is best.

—Avoid using multiple fonts or multiple colors.

—Underline or circle key points.

Examples of patient-friendly materials can be seen in the case study of St Luke's Hospital, Cedar Rapids, Iowa, in a *How-to Guide for Reducing Avoidable Readmissions*. This guide assists hospital staff to improve patient safety in transitions out of hospitals.[19]

• Create a patient literacy panel that reviews educational materials and processes used in the organization. (*See* Sidebar 9-5, page 100.) Members can include nurses, patient safety professionals, and patients. Try to include two or more representatives of persons with low literacy, so your organization can assess whether the materials are appropriate for most patients. Policies could include a provision to invite individuals with low health literacy to edit patient education materials by striking through words that they do not understand to identify areas that need alternative plain language wording.

• Incorporate effective teaching methods for patients. This involves making education relevant and easy to understand and confirming patient understanding. As with written material, providers should use simple terms and short statements when speaking with patients and avoid complicated medical jargon. Providers should slow down and give patients ample time to ask questions and express concerns. Other strategies include the following:

—Use the teach-back method to confirm patient understanding.[20] This approach involves providers asking

---

---

patients to state in their own words (teach-back) key concepts, decisions, or instructions just discussed. If a patient can restate your instructions correctly, then the patient education you provided was effective. If not, then you need to explain the instructions again, using simple words and additional methods of education, such as pictures, brochures, or demonstrations. The teach-back method can be repeated until you confirm the patient understands your message. If after two or three tries the patient still does not demonstrate understanding, then look for other explanations (beyond your teaching) about why the message is not understood. For patients who do not understand your message, the next step might be to give a referral to a patient educator, encourage the patient to bring a family member or friend to the next appointment, or make an appointment for a follow-up visit or phone call.[21]

Care must be taken when using the teach-back method so that it is done in a nonshaming way. Frame the discussion in a way that does not imply that the patient didn't understand. For example, saying "I want to confirm that I've done a good job teaching" may be helpful. Another approach may be to say, "I know your family is coming today. What do you plan to say to them about our session today?"

Consider ways to improve competence in the use of teach-back, which may include having staff practice with, observe, and coach one another. Things to look for in teaching and use of teach-back include use of plain language and simple, understandable terms and analogies; the request for teach-back asks for a response in the patient's own words; use of nonshaming language; friendly body language and tone of voice and attitude; and avoidance of questions with "yes" or "no" answers.

—Encourage patients to Ask Me 3™, which empowers them to ask and know the answers to three main concepts every time education is provided[22]:

1. What is my main problem?
2. What do I need to do?
3. Why is it important for me to do this?

In addition to encouraging patients to ask these three questions, providers are encouraged to teach to these questions as well. For example, when teaching patients about falls and why it is important for them to call and ask for assistance when going to the bathroom, the provider should take the following approach:

1. What's my main problem? You are at risk for falling, particularly on the way to the bathroom, because of the new medicine you began taking today.

2. What should I do for that main problem? When you need to go to the bathroom, call me using this call button here. Let me show you how to use it.

3. Why is it important? Because if you fall you could get hurt and we want to keep you from getting hurt.

At the close of the teaching, providers should use teach-back to confirm that the patient understood what was taught and can use the call light to call the nurse. For example, you could say to the patient, "Your husband is coming to visit today. Could you please tell me what you are going to tell him about the need to get help to the bathroom?" As the patient teaches back, the provider can identify gaps and teach to the gaps.

In addition to helping ensure that patients receive the appropriate education, the Ask Me 3 program can play an important role in creating a shame-free environment, show that questions are welcomed and expected, help make

Figure 9-1. Ask Me 3™

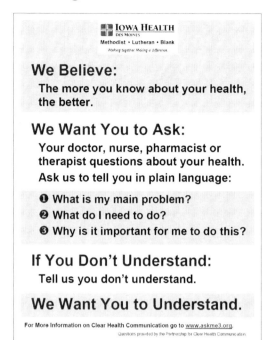

Iowa Health uses this flyer to help educate patients on the Ask Me 3 program.

Source: Iowa Health System. Used with permission.

patients feel more comfortable, and enhance communication with providers. Exemplar organizations in patient experience have noted a link between patients' comfort with speaking up and higher patient experience results.[23] (Figure 9-1, above, shows one organization's education tools for the Ask Me 3 approach.)

—Use return demonstration. "Return demonstration" or "show back" is another patient education method in which the patient is asked to demonstrate to the caregiver how he or she will do what was taught. This technique is used routinely in diabetic education and physical therapy.[24]

—Segment complex education. When patients require complex care and thus multifaceted education—such as with cardiac care or cancer treatment—you may want to break down education into manageable chunks and prioritize when specific information is taught. For example, in cardiac care, the first session may cover important medica-

tions and how patients can weigh themselves. After the patient is comfortable with this topic, a subsequent session may focus on diet and exercise. At the conclusion of each segment, providers should use teach-back to verify patient understanding and ask what additional questions the patient may have.

—When designing and implementing revised patient education materials and teaching methods, establish performance measures to determine the success of these initiatives. Some of these measures may include the number of unplanned admissions, missed appointments, repeat visits, and medication errors.

—Partner across the care continuum to redesign patient education and give patients consistent messages, teaching, and written materials. Methods demonstrating how cross-continuum teams can work together to engage patients and families in design of safer transitions process are described elsewhere.[24] Review methods used to educate and create awareness for patients/families to be involved. Is it part of the admission process? What vital self-care information needs to be taught in the hospital and what should be taught in subsequent care settings when it is easier for patients to take in new information?

—Be aware that transitions of care, such as discharge, are critical times to engage patients and help ensure that they understand the process of their care. In addition, patients/families should be asked to assess their perception of the care experience. Simple questions such as, "What did we do well? What could we have done better? What would you like to see the next time?" demonstrate that the organization cares, and they afford an opportunity to gather ideas for further improvement.

SUMMARY

Partnering with patients and families is an important part of fostering an organizational culture that supports ongoing improvement in patient safety. Involving them in all aspects of care, respecting their preferences and beliefs, and engaging in conversations and discussions to understand the unique needs of each individual patient will lead to safer care and a better overall patient experience.

REFERENCES

1. Dana-Farber Cancer Institute. Establishing Patient- and Family-Centered Care. Accessed Oct 31, 2012. http://www.dana-farber.org/Adult-Care/New-Patient-Guide/Adult-Patient-and-Family-Advisory-Council/Establishing-Patient-and-Family-Centered-Care.aspx.

2. The Joint Commission. *2012 Comprehensive Accreditation Manual for Hospitals: The Official Handbook.* Oak Brook, IL: Joint Commission Resources, 2011.

3. Schillinger D, et al. Closing the loop: Physician communication with diabetic patients who have low health literacy. *Arch Intern Med.* 2003 Jan 13;163(1):83–90.

4. Fahey L, Schilling L. Nurse knowledge exchange: Patient hand offs. *AAACN Viewpoint.* 2007;(5):6–8.

5. Rudd RE, Anderson JE. *The Health Literacy Environment of Hospitals and Health Centers: Partners for Action: Making Your Healthcare Facility Literacy-Friendly.* Boston: Harvard School of Public Health, National Center for the Study of Adult Learning and Literacy Health, 2006. Accessed Oct 31, 2012. http://www.hsph.harvard.edu/healthliteracy/files/healthliteracyenvironment.pdf.

6. Agency for Healthcare Research and Quality. TeamSTEPPS®: National Implementation. Accessed Oct 31, 2012. http://teamstepps.ahrq.gov/.

7. Institute for Patient- and Family-Centered Care. Changing Hospital "Visiting" Policies and Practices: Supporting Family Presence and Participation. Oct 2010. Accessed Oct 31, 2012. http://www.ipfcc.org/visiting.pdf.

8. Planetree, Picker Institute. Patient-Centered Care Improvement Guide: Practical Approaches for Building a Patient-Centered Culture. Accessed Oct 31, 2012. http://www.patient-centeredcare.org/inside/practical.html#F.

9. Nielsen-Bohlman L, Panzer AM, Kindig DA, editors; Committee on Health Literacy, Institute of Medicine. *Health Literacy: A Prescription to End Confusion.* Washington, DC: National Academies Press, 2004.

10. Berkman ND, et al. *Health Literacy Interventions and Outcomes: An Updated Systematic Review.* Evidence Report/Technology Assessment No. 199. Rockville, MD: Agency for Healthcare Research and Quality, Mar 2011. Accessed Oct 31, 2012. http://www.ahrq.gov/downloads/pub/evidence/pdf/literacy/literacyup.pdf.

11. Ratzan SC, Parker RM. Introduction. In Selden CR, et al., editors: *US National Library of Medicine: Current Bibliographies in Medicine: Health Literacy.* NLM Pub. No. CBM 2000-1. Bethesda, MD: National Institutes of Health, US Department of Health & Human Services, 2000, v–vi.

12. Kutner M, et al. *The Health Literacy of America's Adults: Results from the 2003 National Assessment of Adult Literacy.* NCES Pub. No. 2006-483. Washington, DC: US Department of Education, National Center for Education Statistics, 2006. Accessed Oct 31, 2012. http://nces.ed.gov/naal/health.asp.

13. Parikh NS, et al. Shame and health literacy: The unspoken connection. *Patient Educ Couns.* 1996;27(1):33–39.

14. Weiss BD. *Health Literacy and Patient Safety: Help Patients Understand: Manual for Clinicians,* 2nd ed. Chicago: American Medical Association Foundation, 2007.

15. George Washington University. Low Health Literacy: Implications for National Health Policy. Vernon J, et al. Oct 2007. Accessed Oct 31, 2012. http://sphhs.gwu.edu/departments/healthpolicy/dhp_publications/pub_uploads/dhpPublication_3AC9A1C2-5056-9D20-3D4BC6786DD46B1B.pdf

16. American Medical Association Foundation. *Health Literacy and Patient Safety: Help Patients Understand: Reducing the Risk by Designing a Safer, Shame-Free Health Care Environment.* Chicago: American Medical Association Foundation, Aug 2007. Accessed Jul 19, 2012. http://www.ama-assn.org/ama1/pub/upload/mm/367/hl_monograph.pdf.

17. Koh HK, et al. New federal policy initiatives to boost health literacy can help the nation move beyond the cycle of costly 'crisis care'. *Health Aff (Millwood).* 2012;31(2):434-43. Accessed Oct 31, 2012. http://content.healthaffairs.org/content/early/2012/01/18/hlthaff.2011.1169.

18. DeWalt DA, et al. *Health Literacy Universal Precautions Toolkit.* AHRQ Pub. No. 10-0046-EF. Rockville, MD: Agency for Healthcare Research and Quality, Apr 2010. Accessed Oct 31, 2012. http://www.ahrq.gov/qual/literacy/healthliteracytoolkit.pdf.

19. Schall M, et al. *How-to Guide: Improving Transitions from the Hospital to the Clinical Office Practice to Reduce Avoidable Rehospitalizations.* Cambridge, MA: Institute for Healthcare Improvement, Jun. 2012. Accessed Oct 31, 2012. http://www.ihi.org/knowledge/Pages/Tools/HowtoGuideImprovingTransitionsHospitaltoOfficePracticeReduceRehospitalizations.aspx.

20. Schillinger D, et al. Closing the loop: Physician communication with diabetic patients who have low health literacy. *Arch Intern Med.* 2003 Jan 13;163(1):83–90. Accessed Oct 31, 2012. http://archinte.ama-assn.org/cgi/content/full/163/1/83.

21. Health Literacy Consulting. In Other Words . . . Confirming Understanding with the Teach-Back Technique. Osborne H. Accessed Oct 31, 2012. http://www.healthliteracy.com/article.asp?PageID=6714

22. National Patient Safety Foundation. Ask Me 3. Accessed Oct 31, 2012. http://www.npsf.org/askme3/.

23. Personal communication between the author [B.B.] and Kristine White, Vice President, Innovation and Patient Affairs, Spectrum Health System, Grand Rapids, MI, Oct 2011.

24. Nielsen GA, et al. *Transforming Care at the Bedside How-to Guide: Creating an Ideal Transition Home for Patients with Heart Failure.* Cambridge, MA: Institute for Healthcare Improvement, 2008. Accessed Oct 31, 2012. http://www.ihi.org/knowledge/Pages/Tools/TCABHowToGuideTransitionHomeforHF.aspx.

Chapter Ten

USING TECHNOLOGY TO ENHANCE SAFETY

Jeffrey P. Brown, MEd; Jackie Tonkel, BSBA; David C. Classen, MD, MS

Historically, information technology has been used in health care almost exclusively for financial and administrative activities. This is no longer the case. In the United States, the Health Information Technology for Economic and Clinical Health (HITECH) Act—federal legislation that is part of the American Recovery and Reinvestment Act (ARRA) of 2009—offers nearly $30 billion in financial incentives for hospitals and practitioners to adopt certified electronic health records (EHRs) and use them in meaningful ways.[1-3] This legislation has spurred wide adoption of health information technology (HIT) in actual patient care across the continuum,[1-3] which has clearly begun to influence patient safety. With respect to the Institute of Medicine (IOM), for virtually all its patient safety reports in the last 15 years, information technology has been viewed as key to safer patient care, and, in its 2011 report *Health IT and Patient Safety: Building Safer Systems for Safer Care*, is now front and center.[1] In this chapter, we review the current state of HIT as it relates to health care delivery and discuss how HIT can and will be used to both measure and improve patient safety.[4]

CURRENT STATE OF HEALTH CARE INFORMATION TECHNOLOGY
Diversity of Definitions of HIT

Traditionally, HIT was viewed as consisting of electronic health records (EHRs; also termed *electronic medical records*) systems in hospitals or clinics, and the increased adoption of HIT during the last five years has been largely in EHRs in those settings and elsewhere across the continuum of care. However, many other aspects of health care have also been the focus of automation, including billing and claim systems; radiology systems; communication systems; and medical devices, such as monitors and remote monitoring sensors. For the purpose of this chapter, HIT is defined broadly, as in the 2011 IOM report,[1] to include any system that facilitates patient care across the continuum—EHR systems; patient engagement tools such as remote monitoring or personal health records (PHRs), which allow patients access to their medical record information; and Health Information Exchange (HIE) systems and their spin-offs—but not regulated medical devices, such as intravenous pumps or ventilators.

Health Information Technology Adoption

Adoption of all forms of HIT has grown significantly during the last 10 years in the United States, with the greatest growth in EHRs. Most hospitals now have a basic EHR system, as do more than 50% of physician practices, reflecting the influence of federal incentives.[2-3] In addition, HIEs—entities that facilitate the exchange of patient information between health care organizations (and that did not exist 20 years ago)—are now commonplace in many large metropolitan areas. Although the lack of a clear business case has made many HIEs dependent on grants or subsidies,[2,3] they have become a major presence in health care, allowing for patient information to be widely shared among a panoply of providers and providing the infrastructure needed to support the medical home concept and many functions of accountable care organizations. Both public and private HIEs exist and will be a key part of patient care during the years to come.

PHRs were introduced almost 10 years ago with great fanfare, but many leading PHR vendors have subsequently left the marketplace. Although the future role of stand-alone

PHRs remains unclear, PHRs linked to EHRs are commonplace and growing. The use of other patient engagement tools, such as remote patient monitoring systems and patient portals, is also increasing, and such tools may have a far greater impact than stand-alone PHR systems.[1]

HIT and Meaningful Use

The HITECH Act's financial incentives have attracted significant interest on the part of hospitals, most of which appear to be planning to meet the relevant criteria for the incentives, which, for a 250-bed hospital, for example, can amount to millions of dollars. The incentives for practitioners, which can total more than $40,000, have also attracted much interest. Although actual official meaningful use attestation remains low, it is growing rapidly on the part of hospitals and practitioners.[1-3] The meaningful use incentives have been broken into three stages over multiple years, with the criteria for the first phase finalized and those for the second stage recently finalized; criteria for the third stage remain to be elucidated.[3] Many of the criteria in the first two stages are driven by patient safety improvement goals, such as those related to the use of computerized provider order entry (CPOE), medication reconciliation, decision support, exchange of clinical information, and the tracking of patient safety and quality metrics. EHR vendors have enhanced their products to meet meaningful use criteria and achieve meaningful use certification, which is required for hospitals or practitioners to attest with a vendor product that is officially certified.[1]

HIT National Data Standards

One of the challenges in improving safety with EHRs is achieving the interoperability of HIT systems necessary for the free flow of critical patient information. To facilitate this goal, previous IOM reports have called for the national adoption of HIT standards—including those addressing the laboratory, such as Logical Observation Identifiers Names and Codes (LOINC®); imaging, such as Digital Imaging and Communications in Medicine (DICOM); vocabulary, such as RX Norm; and disease classifications, such as Systematized Nomenclature of Medicine—Clinical Terms (SNOMED Clinical Terms®).[5] Meaningful use certification requires that vendors adopt these standards or risk being decertified.[5] In terms of patient safety, a similar movement is forthcoming as part of the Patient Safety Organization legislation allowing for standard patient safety classifications using Agency for Healthcare Research and Quality common formats. These formats have been developed with specific HIT specifications to enable the automation of this content in electronic systems.[6,7] These patient safety classifications will form the basis for initial patient safety standards within HIT.[7]

LOOKING FORWARD: PATIENT SAFETY AND HIT—THE IOM REPORT

The first part of *Health IT and Patient Safety*[1] outlines the current state of patient safety more than 12 years after the landmark IOM report *To Err Is Human,* which stated that as many as 98,000 patients may die every year in hospitals in the United States from patient safety problems.[8] As cited in the 2011 IOM report,[1] an Office of the Inspector General study of hospitalized Medicare patients suggests that as many as 180,000 hospitalized Medicare patients may die every year as a result of hospital-acquired adverse events.[9] This estimate does not include the non-Medicare hospital populations, so the true number of hospital-related deaths from patient safety problems may be as high as several hundred thousand per year. This sets a new level of harm in the health care system, despite more than a decade of work to improve patient safety. In the setting of this new level of harm in the system, the increased efforts to improve patient safety will increasingly involve technology, with increasingly rapid HIT adoption changing the landscape of health care.[1]

HIT–Caused Harm

Given these new harm estimates, the need for HIT that actually improves the safety of care is great, but with the greater visibility of HIT associated with large financial incentives, the risk of catastrophic HIT accidents also looms large. The first rule of health care is do no harm. The 2011 IOM report outlines several incidents in which HIT has directly lead to patient injury or death. However, it underlines the reality that most safety tracking systems underreport safety problems in general, and HIT safety problems in particular, so that the true incidence of HIT safety issues is unknown. In addition, many HIT vendors have contractual limitations that prevent users from publicly sharing safety problems, and there is no effective government safety tracking system for this largely unregulated industry.[1]

HIT–Reduced Harm

Many of the reports advocating the HITECH Act and the associated meaningful use criteria based their approach on previously published studies outlining the safety benefits of HIT. However, many of those studies come from health care organizations with internally developed ("home-grown") HIT systems rather than the commercial HIT systems that are now in widespread use. On balance, the 2011 IOM report says that the benefits of HIT are best demonstrated in medication safety but poorly demonstrated in other areas of safety, with competing conclusions from various studies. Moreover, HIT can play a key role in improving the detection of all safety problems and not just those safety issues related to HIT.[1]

CHALLENGES IN IMPROVING SAFETY WITH HIT

One of the challenges in improving safety with HIT is that the few studies performed that have measured the safety of HIT systems in actual routine operation have found large deficiencies in critical safety checks for medication safety alone, which is usually the most sophisticated patient safety intervention in most EHR systems.[10] As the report explains, this is not unexpected, in that other industries have learned that complex systems continually test and refine operation systems to improve safety performance, as well as build human factors and cognitive engineering concepts into the systems from ground zero. This has not been accomplished in most HIT systems to date but will need to be present in future systems.[1]

Patient and Family Utilization of HIT

Patient-/family-centered care, which reflects the belief that health care providers and families are partners, working together to best meet the needs of patients and the patients' families, is heavily emphasized in the IOM report as a critical requirement to improve the safety of care.[1] One goal of the EHR incentive program for meaningful use is the engagement of patients and their families in patients' health care. This policy aims to improve patients' understanding of their health and related conditions so they take a more active role in their health care. It also encourages the involvement of patients' families, on whom many patients depend for support. The use of certified EHR technologies can assist in making health information more readily available to both families and providers. Meaningful use of EHRs will also enable providers to involve patients and their families in more informed decision-making while promoting patients' management of their own health.[1]

Excellence in health care happens when providers and patients and their families work together and honor the expertise that everyone brings to every health encounter. Patient-/family-centered care represents a continual effort to be responsive to the needs and choices of each family, and meaningful use criteria are intended to help support the relevant information sharing necessary to make appropriate health care decisions.

How can meaningful use affect patient-centeredness and engagement? A key focus of meaningful use is interoperability. It is believed that its standards and requirements will help ensure a common language to allow for accurate and secure health information exchange among providers and families. Informed and educated patients and their families can take a more active role in health care decision making, especially when having to choose among multiple treatment options. Having access to information, education materials, and other tools can help patients and their families participate in treatment decisions with providers. In addition, having patients more involved can have a substantial impact on their overall health, especially as it relates to chronic diseases such as diabetes and asthma that require self-management.[1]

Better use of health care resources is an additional benefit of patient-centered care supported by meaningful use, as represented, for example, by a patient with cancer who needs to see multiple care providers before receiving treatment. Electronic access to medical records, laboratory tests, procedures, and x-rays can reduce the need for redundant testing or procedures and eliminate the need for patients and their families to carry around (and possibly lose) important health records and documentation. Meaningful use, which is intended to help measurably improve quality, safety, and the cost of health care, in the context of patient and family engagement, is intended to help provide patients and families with access to data, knowledge, and tools to make informed decisions and to manage their health.[1]

HEALTH CARE IS A SOCIOTECHNICAL ENDEAVOR

On the basis of the concepts presented in the previous section, the 2011 IOM report outlined a series of steps to increase the transparency of HIT vendor performance and called for HIT vendors to adopt quality management processes. Reporting of safety problems, with a focus on both voluntary reporting and surveillance, was a key part of the report. Drawing from aviation, the report recommended a National Transportation Safety Board–like approach to collect, analyze, and investigate patient safety problems related to HIT, something quite unusual for health care. Finally, it called for Food and Drug Administration (FDA) regulation of HIT if industry self-regulation fails to improve HIT safety.[1]

The IOM report also recommended a new conceptual framework for understanding and managing HIT and patient safety—the Sociotechnical System Model. The diversity of roles, tasks, and process interdependencies among people, environments, and technologies mark health care systems as socially and technologically complex; they are complex *sociotechnical systems.* Health care systems may also be characterized as "high-consequence," given that they carry the risk of harm to patients and care providers in event of failure.[11] The continuing occurrence of high levels of patient harm, as discussed earlier, suggests that common approaches to the improvement and measurement of patient safety are not yet sufficient to move health care systems from "low reliability" to "high reliability."

The Sociotechnical System Model is depicted in Figure 10-1 (at right).

As described in the IOM report, the components of the Sociotechnical Model are as follows:

Technology includes the hardware and software of HIT, which are organized and developed under an architecture that specifies and delivers the functionality required from different parts of HIT, as well as how these different parts interact with each other. From the perspective of health professionals, technology can also include more clinically based information (for example, order sets), although technologists regard order sets as the responsibility of clinical experts.

People relates to individuals working within the entire sociotechnical system, including their knowledge and skills regarding both clinical work and technology. It also includes their cognitive capabilities, such as memory, inferential strategies, and knowledge. In addition to these individual aspects, the "people" component encompasses the implementation teams that configure and support the technology and those who train clinical users. Technology has an impact

Figure 10-1. Sociotechnical System Underlying HIT–Related Adverse Events

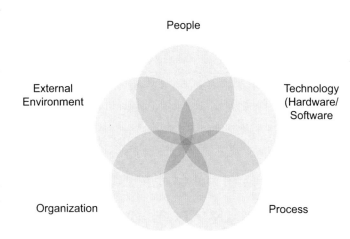

Source: Committee on Patient Safety and *Health Information Technology, Institute of Medicine. Health IT and Patient Safety: Building Safer Systems for Better Care.* Washington, DC: National Academies Press, 2012. [Adapted from Harrington L, Kennerly D, Johnson C. Safety issues related to the electronic medical record (EMR): Synthesis of the literature from the last decade, 2000–2009. *J Healthc Manag.* 2011;56(1):31–44; Sittig DF, Singh H. Eight rights of safe electronic health record use. *JAMA.* 2009 Sep 9;302(10): 1111–1113; Walker JM, et al. EHR safety: The way forward to safe and effective systems. *J Am Med Inform Assoc.* 2008;15(3):272–277.] Reprinted with permission.

on people; for example, the use of HIT may affect clinician cognition by changing and shaping how clinicians obtain, organize, and analyze information. The way that health care information and data are organized influences the way people solve problems. The scope and nature of clinicians' interactions with technology and with each other in a technology-mediated fashion are very likely to affect clinical outcomes.

Process (sometimes referred to as *work flow*) refers to the normative set of actions and procedures that clinicians are expected to perform during the course of delivering health care. Many of the procedures clinicians use to interact with the technology are prescribed, either formally in documentation (for example, a user's manual, policies and procedures) or informally by the norms and practices of the work environment immediately surrounding the individual. *Process* also includes such tasks as patient scheduling, refilling prescriptions, or ordering diagnostic testing.

Organization refers to organizational decisions relating to technology, including HIT installation, configuration choices, and interfaces with other HIT products. In addition, organizations choose clinical content to be used in HIT. These choices reflect the organization's goals, such as maximizing use of expensive diagnostic equipment, remaining competitive with other health care facilities, and minimizing costs. Of particular relevance is the organization's role in promoting the safety of patient care while maximizing effectiveness and efficiency. *Organization* also includes the internal rules and regulations set by individual institutions, such as hospital policies and procedures that clinicians must follow. In addition, it encompasses the environment in which clinicians work. In many institutions, the environment of care is chaotic and unpredictable—with clinicians frequently interrupted in the course of their day and subject to multiple distractions from patients, coworkers, and others.

External environment refers to the outside influences that affect the way in which health care organizations operate. Federal, state, and private-sector entities (such as accreditation organizations and third-party payers) establish rules and regulations that dictate how health care organizations and providers operate. For example, health care organizations are required to publicly report on predetermined measures of quality, including errors made in the course of providing care, failure to follow established standards of care, and rates of infections.

COMPONENT-CENTERED VERSUS SYSTEM-BASED SAFETY MANAGEMENT

Findings from research across high-consequence industries suggest that poor progress made in the improvement of patient safety may be due, in substantial part, to the approach to safety management employed by health care organizations.[12] Typically, patient safety improvement strategies focus on enhancing the reliability of components of health care delivery systems. For example, checklists may enhance the reliability of task preparation and performance, wrist bands may remind staff of certain patient conditions/risks, smart infusion pumps may help prevent inappropriate dosing of medication, failure mode and effects analysis may be applied for the improvement of a patient care process, or the layout of a clinical unit may be designed with the intention of enhancing communication and coor-

dination. Although such efforts to create high-reliability organizations that ensure the reliable performance of people, technologies, and processes are necessary, a focus on individual system components does not adequately support the organization in detecting, identifying, and mitigating unanticipated adverse effects stemming from *component interactions*. The case in Sidebar 10-1 (*see* page 108) underscores the IOM's call for an approach to safety assessment and risk mitigation that illuminates the emergent effects of interaction among people, technology, processes, organization, and environment.

As described in Sidebar 10-1, implementation of HIT in an emergency department (ED) altered communication and coordination, undermining the quality and safety of patient care and incurring significant inefficiency. Conducting a study of human, process, technological, environmental, and organizational component interactions in the unit to be served by HIT, which can help identify and mitigate potential adverse HIT implementation effects, is necessary in advance of both selection and implementation.[13] Postimplementation surveillance and investigation of unintended effects on system performance are also needed. The problems illustrated by the case in Sidebar 10-1 might not have been addressed as quickly if patient satisfaction scores had not garnered the attention of the CEO. Before the "all hands" meeting, a growing collection of patient complaints and a handful of safety reports caught the attention of the quality, patient safety, and risk management offices (these were considered separate, rather than integrated, functions). The investigation of the patient complaints led to a recommendation for a refresher on a [theme park–based] training program on customer service, and new posters were tacked up in the staff break room promoting "Excellence in Patient Care." Investigation of the safety reports led to the finding that nurses were not responding to physicians' orders on a timely basis—without considering why this might be. This resulted in the requirement that nurses receive reeducation on nursing policy and procedure, and the ED nurse supervisor was also advised to counsel nurses identified in incident reports regarding their performance and to set improvement goals. In effect, this initiated a progressive disciplinary process. None of these actions addressed the underlying conditions for failure that emerged from the interaction of clinical personnel, unit-level organization, the clinical environment, and extant care

---

Sidebar 10-1. Case: Communication and Coordination Deficit Introduced with the Implementation of Health Information Technology

We implemented [an information technology system] in our emergency department (ED). Within a few weeks of implementation the climate of our ED had changed; the physicians were complaining that nurses weren't on top of their orders. And nurses and technicians were complaining that doctors weren't communicating their orders and intentions with them anymore. Our patient satisfaction went into the hopper because of delays and suboptimal care. This got the CEO's attention because his pay is linked to patient satisfaction. We had an urgent 'all hands' ED meeting to figure out how we had gotten in such a mess and what we needed to do to get patient satisfaction scores up.

It turns out that we all thought we could see each other's notes in the computer, but we couldn't. Information that used to be said out loud was no longer spoken, just entered into the computer. We used to depend on hearing orders and updates—even if we just overheard—to anticipate patients' needs and coordinate our work. It was a big part how each of us knew what was going on and could backup each other and the care processes.

Ironically, [the HIT vendor] marketed the system by asserting that it would improve coordination, efficiency, and patient safety in the ED! We're still trying to figure out how to make the information system work for us. For now, we are making sure to verbally communicate everything we enter into the computer. It's inefficient, but necessary.

Source: Jeffrey P. Brown. Used with permission.

---

processes with the new HIT system. Rather, the focus was on people; specifically, the ways in which nurses were not complying with policy and procedure. Interaction with the new information technology in the clinical context was not considered.

The foregoing case raises a number of questions, beginning with "How can hospitals better implement and monitor information technology?" Assessment of sociotechnical systems, using, for example, ethnography and cognitive work analysis methods, before selecting and implementing information technology can reveal process constraints, information requirements, and goal conflicts and the tacit strategies employed by clinicians to manage them. Aside from illuminating opportunities for immediate improvement, these insights are useful in considering how a candidate information technology may fit into the work flow and how it may serve the information requirements of clinicians. Moreover, after a technology is selected, a better-informed implementation strategy becomes possible, and the same methods used for the initial assessment may be applied to monitor for the emergence of unintended/unanticipated effects of the information technology implementation.

The case also shows how safety or failure in complex systems may be thought of as an "emergent" system property insofar as it stems from interdependencies, interrelationships, and interactions among the components of the system rather than from the failure of a single element.[13] These components routinely interact not only across levels and units

within organizations, but in the external environment, across organizations. From a bird's-eye view, these interactions occur across all levels of the health care system in the United States, which may be viewed as a system of systems. This nationwide macro-level encompasses all the medical facilities, regulatory and accreditation entities, regional environments, and regional populations that provide, oversee, contain, or use health care. At the micro-level, a health care delivery system can be thought of as a grouping of people, processes, and technologies organized within a clinical environment to provide care to a specific patient population.[14] Systems and subsystems, from macro-scale to micro-scale, have the same fundamental components—people, technology, organization, process, and environment. "Cross-scale" interactions among these system components are often asynchronous and their effects insidious, going unnoticed for long periods of time. This makes it impossible for individuals, groups, or organizations to anticipate and identify all ways in which their performance may be compromised by the state of distant or otherwise unobservable roles, functions, technologies, and processes. In work domains where personnel cannot directly observe or monitor the processes on which they depend, decisions are made and actions taken with a high degree of uncertainty.

System designers and frontline personnel respond to the risk and uncertainty that is resident in complex systems by attempting to anticipate potential modes of failure and developing safeguards and countermeasures to combat them, such as checklists or smart infusion pumps, as mentioned earlier—or alerts and alarms, redundant operational systems, standard operating procedures, and team/crew training. In addition, frontline operators develop tacit rules and practices to work around problematic features of technology, environment, work processes, and individual, group, and organizational dynamics. For example, regarding a failed medication-dispensing unit on an ICU, a nurse stated the following: "The biometric scanner on our [medication-dispensing] unit is not reliable. When we need medications from the [medication-dispensing unit], we usually need them in a hurry. We reported the problem multiple times, got no action, and then gave up. We just run [literally] to the satellite pharmacy rather than take the chance of wasting time."

Such work-arounds emerge as clinicians strive to avoid the failures and/or inefficiencies based on problematic experience. Frontline work-arounds may be seen as a symptom of deeper problems in the system—commonly involving both local and cross-scale component interaction. In this case, multiple influences were implicated in the "normalization" of the nurses' work-around, including maintenance requests that did not convey urgency; a staffing reduction in the biomedical engineering department, which delayed response to maintenance requests; and an organizational and professional culture that held personnel accountable for getting things done with the resources at hand.

Although work-arounds make it possible to accomplish work in the face of constraints, they may also pose risk. As related by an ICU nurse, the nursing staff stopped reporting the unreliable biometric scanner when they perceived that no corrective response was forthcoming and rapidly normalized their work-around. The risk associated with delay in obtaining critical medications, whether due to malfunction of the medication-dispensing unit or having to run to the satellite pharmacy, remained resident and effectively invisible to the organization. An important insight for patient safety officers, illustrated by the case, is that if there are impediments to the communication of risk by frontline personnel and to obtaining rapid organizational response, work-arounds will become "normalized" quickly, rendering them invisible to risk and safety personnel—they will fly "under the radar." Patient safety officers must remain vigilant for signs of change in frontline practice that may signal the emergence of a work-around and the need for risk assessment.

Although the risk associated with some adaptations and work-arounds may not be immediately obvious, the following case, as reported by a physician patient safety executive (Sidebar 10-2, page 110), illustrates how frontline adaptations/work-arounds may quickly manifest as an unsafe, emergent effect of interaction among system components.[10] This case illustrates how changes that are initiated, and perceived as innocuous, at one system level may significantly and unexpectedly compromise functionality and safety at another. The morphine administration process became unworkable in the context of busy, clinical work as a side-effect of executive decision making. Executive decision making and governance decision making (the impetus for cost-cutting came from the board of directors in this case), clearly can have a direct impact on the safety and quality of clinical care.

A striking feature of this case is the unintended subversion of the safety purposes of bar coding in medication administration technology as a result of changing a single drug from a bar-coded to a non–bar-coded product. Again, technologies cast as safety "solutions" can quickly be undone by unanticipated, cross-scale interactions among system components. The reliability and safety of technology clearly is not all about the design of software and hardware. In health care and other high-risk, high-consequence domains, accidents may be seen as the end product of a cascade of decision side effects that often have their beginnings at the governance and executive levels. It is important for patient safety officers to promote the participation of board members and senior executives in their organization's patient safety committee. In this way, those with authority to redress a safety issue—that has emerged as a side effect of executive decision making—can be directly involved in both the analysis and development of a corrective response.

CONSIDERATIONS FOR SYSTEM-BASED SAFETY MANAGEMENT

Understanding the effects of implementing or altering technology, whether for improvement in the quality and safety of patient care or for other purposes, requires new, research-based approaches to the design, development, implementation, and optimization of systems of care. Pending these advances, a key challenge for patient safety officers is to promote a system-based perspective on safety in their organizations. We now provide some considerations for this purpose.

Sidebar 10-2. Frontline Adaptations/Work-Arounds Can Undermine Patient Safety

Our risk management office advised me that a nurse educator wanted help. Syringes containing morphine were being found in the clinical areas of the hospital. There are laws, policies, and procedures to prevent this, and the nurse educator's effort to stop the problem through education and admonition had no effect. I was very concerned and curious because this was a previously unheard of problem in our organization.

On exploring the issue with the nurse educator, I learned that nurses had begun keeping syringes with morphine solution in their pockets or were putting the syringes down before wasting the excess and then forgetting to come back and finish the wasting process.

I went to the floor and teamed with a nurse to walk through the medication administration process. We looked at a patient's chart, which had an order to administer 4 mg morphine every two hours. We then went to the medication dispenser, a secure box with narcotics and drugs prescribed for the patient for each day. To access the drugs, the nurse entered her identification and opened the dispenser. Inside was a 10 mg ampoule of morphine. The nurse informed me that this was now the only size carried in our pharmacy. It was also the only non–bar-coded medication in our pharmacy. I learned that a decision had been made by the vice president who oversees pharmacy to stop purchasing bar-coded doses of morphine and to purchase the 10 mg, non–bar-coded morphine because it's cheaper. There was a big cost-reduction initiative in the organization—although morphine is relatively cheap, so I don't know why it was specifically selected among all other bar-coded medications. Although this change in purchasing might not seem like a big deal, it had significant impact on nursing work processes.

Because nurses do not use 10 mg of morphine at once, they must go to a separate area, draw the needed amount into a syringe, and dilute it to 1 mg per cc. Then they look for a bar code scanner to "tell" it they are going to dose the patient. However, they can't just scan in the information because these morphine vials have no bar code. Nurses have to override the bar code function and enter that they are administering only 4 mg, not 10 mg. Once that's accomplished, they find a handheld scanner and scan the patient's armband to tell the device they are about to administer the morphine and then that it has been delivered. After that, they must find another nurse to witness them dispose of the excess morphine. Finally, they document the patient's response to the injection.

The morphine administration process had become incredibly time consuming, intruding on other patient care needs and responsibilities. Not surprisingly, if a nurse was unable to find another nurse to witness the disposal of excess morphine and a patient needed attention, the syringe would go into his or her pocket, or get put down for disposal later (if remembered). Then nurses just began saving the syringe for the next shot to avoid the entire rigmarole.

The added steps and delays that were introduced by a switch to non–bar-coded morphine undermined the ability of nurses to meet the needs of their patients, complete other duties, and ultimately provoked a hazardous work-around. By the way, we had a shortage of bar code scanners and were dealing with a nursing shortage when the change in morphine purchasing hit. It was a perfect storm of contributing factors.

Source: Adapted from Brown JP. Achieving high reliability: Other industries can help health care's safety transformation. *Journal of Healthcare Risk Management.* 2004;24(2):15–25. Copyright © 2004 John Wiley & Sons. Reproduced with permission of John Wiley & Sons, Inc.

People Are the Core Source of System Resilience and Safety

If work-arounds are a symptom of systemic problems, as has been argued, experience across multiple high-risk domains has also demonstrated that effective management of uncertainty and risk in complex systems hinges on the ability of people to detect anomalies or problems, to identify and make sense of emergent situations, and adapt activity and action to maintain or restore safety and system functionality.[15–17] Although they are rarely characterized this way, a central purpose of training programs aimed at improving clinical team processes is to enhance the ability of small frontline groups to detect, identify, mitigate, and recover from emergent problems. Interprofessional clinical teams, because of their varied expertise and perspectives, have the potential to become very adept at problem detection, analysis, and resolution.[18–20] The following statement by Weick can help us to understand why:

> When technical systems have more variety than a single individual can comprehend, one of the few ways humans can match this variety is by networks and teams of divergent individuals. . . . Whether team members differ in occupational specialties, past experience, gender, conceptual skills, or personality may be less crucial than the fact that they do differ and look for different things when they size up a problem. If people look for different things, when their observations are pooled they collectively see more than any one of them alone would see.[21(p. 333)]

Historically, system engineering has focused on providing technological controls to protect against system failure and thereby match the potential for component failure with a variety of technological safeguards. The human component was viewed as a source of error and failure that must be countered with technology. The "new view" of the human contribution to system reliability is that the human operator is the one system component that has the capability to resolve the unanticipated forms of failure that emerge in complex systems.[12,22] Identifying design requirements for HIT that will support the clinician in detection and resolution of problems is one factor in enhancing this capability. Another is to organize clinical work to support effective decision making among members of interprofessional frontline teams. Robust team processes support problem detection and resolution, engaging the social element of the sociotechnical system as an adaptive safety mechanism.[19, 23-25] Moreover, insight into the functioning and usability of technology throughout its life cycle can be gathered through routine team debriefing processes. Team debriefing, as a routine practice, remains uncommon in health care. Patient safety officers must continue to lead efforts to develop briefing, debriefing, and other evidence-based team processes in their organizations. Team training, alone, will not ensure development of a high-performing interprofessional team. Observing and characterizing existing team processes in a clinical unit, in advance of team training, enables the patient safety officer to understand how existing technologies, environment, organization, and processes may shape improvement efforts by informing customized requirements for training and implementation design. Working across clinical units permits the patient safety officer to observe and spread useful practices across functional areas of the organization.

HIT Is a Sociotechnical System Component, Prey to the Same Interactive Effects as Other System Components

As we have seen, technology can contribute to emergent safety problems through its interaction with other system components. Yet, the mirror statement is also true—the functionality and safety purposes of technology can be compromised through its interaction with other system components. The sociotechnical perspective views the "system" more broadly than one comprised of software, computer-computer, human-

computer, and human-human interaction. Clinicians do not work alone; they working synchronously and asynchronously with human and machine agents. The provision of patient care is knowledge-intensive, and the information needed to support patient care is voluminous, diverse, and highly distributed. Clinicians continuously "push" and "pull" information, and seek and apply knowledge in support of problem solving, sense making, and decision making. HIT can be a useful adjunct to human-human communication/information exchange, as well as for problem detection, identification, and resolution. However, when design requirements for HIT are predicated on behavioral task analysis, focus groups, preference surveys, and other market research methods, they will reflect an insufficient understanding of both cognitive work and the constraints, goal conflicts, and other behavior-shaping forces that are resident in the system yet largely invisible to its human inhabitants. Even when design requirements for information technologies are reasonably well aligned with the needs of the intended users, changes in the system that alter interaction among its components can undermine functionality, usability, and safety at any time.

HIT implementation should be characterized not as a safety solution but a "safety experiment." Design and implementation hypotheses must be tested in clinical use, for each clinical context of use. Failure Mode and Effects Analysis or other prospective risk identification methods alone are insufficient; implementation of HIT must be accompanied by heightened awareness and monitoring of the potential impact of the technology on overall system functionality, and vice versa. Because the effects of interaction among system components change over time, lasting functionality and system safety can never be assumed. Developing the health care organization's ability to better detect and mitigate emergent risk and safety problems—and to learn from frontline experience—requires significant improvement in system safety surveillance and investigative processes.

Robust Safety Surveillance and Investigation Are the Foundation of Effective Safety Interventions

The challenge of developing effective strategies for assessment of safety in sociotechnical systems is mirrored by the challenge of mitigating risk and improving safety. These challenges exist across high-consequence industries; they are not unique to health care systems. Anticipating all possible forms of failure in complex systems is not possible. The ability to understand failure through postmishap investigation methodologies (root cause analysis, for example) has proven equally problematic; a universal difficulty that derives from efforts to seek an understanding of adverse events or incidents in terms of cause-and-effect relationships.[11] As in other domains, the approach and quality of incident- and adverse-event investigation in health care varies widely both within and across organizations. Methods in common use dwell on component failures that are proximal in time and place to the adverse event—most commonly focusing on people. The process of investigation is typically terminated after a plausible/actionable story of causation is "discovered." More accurately, causation is constructed and is influenced by hindsight bias, counterfactual reasoning, fundamental attribution error, and other well-documented analytical vulnerabilities that may impact the integrity of an investigation.[22] Postinvestigation corrective measures reflect this focus on broken system components. For example, if a patient falls and the bedside care provider hadn't realized the patient was known (by others) to be at risk of fall, a "fix" may be devised that requires a new color-coded "fall risk" placard be applied to the patient's paperwork—"to ensure that everyone knows." Likewise, if a nurse was found to have been noncompliant with a policy or procedure, say, in operating a pump infusion system, the assumption might be that she or he did not understand the policy and procedure associated with the pump, and the resulting remedy might be reeducation on policy and procedure. These approaches typically pay slight attention to the intersection of system influences that create constraints, drive work-arounds, and create failure-provoking conditions. Issues such as porous information flow across units, cultural barriers to unit-level cooperation, hierarchical barriers to risk communication, maintenance deficiencies, awkward technology, unworkable processes, and imbalance between business goals and risk mitigation may go undetected, remaining resident until their effects combine to "bag" another patient and another provider. Fixes aimed at the people found to be closest in time and space to an incident or adverse event routinely omit attention to the underlying and highly distributed factors and forces that may combine to foil even the most skilled and conscientious personnel.

To develop more effective interventions we need to better understand the systemic roots of incidents and adverse events. To this end, the 2011 IOM report recommended use of human factors methodologies not only in the design of HIT but in the implementation, and monitoring of the safety status of HIT in clinical use throughout its life cycle.[1]

Human Factors/Cognitive Systems Engineering Methods Are Essential to Safety Management in Complex Systems

The term *human factors* wraps around many disciplines, including sociology, cognitive psychology, engineering, education, and anthropology, among others. Ultimately, the aim of human factors professionals is to aid in designing tools, processes, technologies, organizations, and environments that support safe and effective human performance. A typical understanding of the relevance of human factors to health care is that it is about developing effective team processes to counter the potential for erroneous action or inaction by individuals through more effective decision making, mutual support, and backup among team members. Another view casts human factors as a discipline that supports the development of design requirements to ensure that technologies, such as HIT, are easy to operate, maintain, and train. Both views are reflected in human factors specializations that address components of the system safety puzzle, not the whole. Human factors professionals, and patient safety officers, working on different pieces of the puzzle, require insight into the functioning of the whole to develop appropriate requirements for its components.

A branch of human factors that has arisen specifically to study and support improvement in sociotechnical systems is called *cognitive systems engineering* (CSE).[26] As described earlier, adverse events typically emerge from the unexpected confluence of component interactions, often when people are performing work the way they usually do to achieve their goals safely and reliably. Yet, how people accomplish work is often quite different in practice than as described in policy and procedure manuals. Over time, constraints and goal conflicts arise as changes occur in task design, financial targets, tools, processes, and other performance-shaping features of the organization and clinical environment. The work-arounds that arise as people adapt to these conflicts and constraints are often not known beyond the clinical unit, and an understanding that an action or activity constitutes a work-around is often quickly lost; becoming "how we do things here." As illustrated by the bar-coding case (Sidebar 10-2), work-arounds and deviations from expected practice may be seen as a manifestation of systemic problems emerging from local and/or cross-scale system interactions. As such, they are useful markers—illuminating points of entry for the investigation of actual work culture, structure, and processes, much as medical contrast media make internal structures of the human body visible, enabling and guiding closer examination. CSE professionals look for these markers in assessing the effectiveness and adaptive capacity of sociotechnical systems and in identifying design requirements for system components.

MAXIMIZING THE BENEFITS OF HIT

Given the sociotechnical system perspective, as we have outlined, and the IOM report's recommendations, what can health care organizations do to begin to operationalize this new approach to HIT? Clearly, HIT offers significant *potential* for improvement in quality, safety, and efficiency. Bates and Kuperman suggest, for example, that EHRs can provide clinicians more timely data access for decision making than paper-based systems and can also organize the data in a way that effectively supports decision making.[4] Similarly, technology can ensure legibility, completeness, and rapid communication with ancillary departments. EHRs in particular can provide clinical decision support, which paper-based medical record systems cannot. Such support may foster standardization, real-time data checking, flags for critical test results, and links to further information and research.[27]

Some of the specific technologies that can improve safety include CPOE; bar coding; smart monitoring, which is monitoring that the computer performs with notification to a provider when appropriate; computerized notification about critical test results; computerized monitoring for adverse drug events; and tracking of abnormal test results.[4] Although the evidence is strongest for improvement of medication safety, HIT can also be helpful for improving handoffs, ensuring that laboratory results receive appropriate follow-up,[1] and, more broadly, for identifying opportunities for improvement in safety and quality.[28]

Yet realizing the benefits of HIT entails overcoming many challenges. Patient safety officers should be aware of these challenges and work to overcome them as they begin to leverage HIT for patient safety improvement. The IOM

sociotechnical system model provides a view of risk and safety that underscores the need to detect and intervene in the unsafe situations that emerge from unanticipated interaction among system components (people, technology, process, environment, and organization). Although there are many tools and tips for patient safety improvement that focus on the *components* of health care systems, there is no research-based "tool box" for identifying and mitigating emergent events. An ongoing and dynamic learning system is essential in devising ways to continually monitor and improve the safety of these systems, and this will necessitate new approaches to safety reporting, investigations, root cause analysis, and conclusions. Koppel et al. have outlined what such an HIT learning system might look like.[29]

CONCLUSION

Health care has often lagged in adopting best practices from other industries. This has certainly been the case with information technology, which until recently had been mainly adopted for billing and financial areas of health care. However, with the passage of the ARRA, and particularly, the HITECH section, which offers financial incentives to implement EHRs, health care is now rushing to implement HIT in clinical care. Yet, as the 2011 IOM report on HIT states, achieving benefits and avoiding risk will require a paradigm change in thinking about health care and HIT, which will entail the use of a sociotechnical model. This model speaks to not only the safe implementation of HIT but the optimization of HIT to achieve maximum safety benefit. HIT implementations need to evolve as safety experiments, with consideration of human factors, cognitive engineering, and the team-based concept to have maximum effect. Applying HIT to the most complex human endeavor of health care will require the development of new approaches for the design, development, implementation, and optimization of the overall system of care, not just information technology.

REFERENCES

1. Committee on Patient Safety and Health Information Technology, Institute of Medicine. *Health IT and Patient Safety: Building Better Systems for Better Care.* Washington, DC: National Academies Press, 2012. Accessed Nov 1, 2012. http://www.iom.edu/Reports/2011/Health-IT-and-Patient-Safety-Building-Safer-Systems-for-Better-Care.aspx.
2. US Department of Health & Human Services, Centers for Medicare & Medicaid Services (CMS): *Electronic Health Record Incentive Program.* Washington, DC: CMS, 2010.

3. Blumenthal D. Implementation of the federal health information technology initiative. *N Engl J Med.* 2011 Dec 22;365(25):2426–2431.

4. Bates DW, Kuperman G. The role of health information technology in quality and safety. In *From Front Office to Front Line: Essential Issues for Health Care Leaders*, 2nd ed. Oak Brook, IL: Joint Commission Resources, 2011, 87–108.

5. Office of the National Coordinator for Health IT (ONC). Certified Health IT Product List. Jun 26, 2012. Accessed Nov 1, 2012. http://onc-chpl.force.com/ehrcert.

6. Agency for Healthcare Research and Quality. Patient Safety and Quality Improvement Act of 2005. Accessed Nov 1, 2012. http://www.pso.ahrq.gov/statute/pl109-41.htm.

7. Clancy CM. Common formats allow uniform collection and reporting of patient safety data by patient safety organizations. *Am J Med Qual.* 2010;25(1):73–75.

8. Institute of Medicine. *To Err Is Human: Building a Better Health System.* Washington, DC: National Academy Press, 2000.

9. US Department of Health & Human Services (DHHS), Office of the Inspector General. *Adverse Events in Hospitals: National Incidence Among Medicare Beneficiaries.* Washington, DC. DHHS, 2010. Accessed Nov 1, 2012. http://oig.hhs.gov/oei/reports/oei-06-09-00090.pdf.

10. Metzger J, et al. Mixed results in the safety performance of computerized physician order entry. *Health Aff (Millwood).* 2010;29(4)655–663.

11. Brown JP. Achieving high reliability: Other industries can help health care's safety transformation. *Journal of Healthcare Risk Management.* 2004;24(2):15–25.

12. Dekker S. *Drift into Failure: From Hunting Broken Components to Understanding Complex Systems.* Farnham, UK: Ashgate, 2011.

13. Woods DD, Hollnagel E. *Joint Cognitive Systems: Patterns in Cognitive Systems Engineering.* Boca Raton, FL: CRC Press, 2006.

14. Nelson, EC, et al. Microsystems in Healthcare: Part 1. Learning from high-performing front-line clinical units. *Jt Comm J Qual Improv.* 2002;28(9):472–493.

15. Klein G, et al. Problem detection. *Cognition, Technology, and Work.* 2005;7(1):14–28.

16. Klein G. The strengths and limitations of teams for detecting problems. *Cognition, Technology, and Work.* 2006;8(4):227–236.

17. Nemeth C. The ability to adapt. In Nemeth CP, Hollnagel E, Dekker S, editors: *Resilience Engineering Perspectives,* vol. 2: *Preparation and Restoration.* Burlington, VT: Ashgate, 2009, 1–12.

18. Bolman LG. Aviation accidents and the theory of the situation. In Cooper GE, editor: *Resource Management on the Flight Deck.* Ames Research Center, Moffett Field, CA: National Aeronautics and Space Administration, 1980, 31–58.

19. Uhlig PN, et al. John M. Eisenberg Patient Safety Awards. System innovation: Concord Hospital. *Jt Comm J Qual Improv.* 2002;28(12):666–672.

20. Nemeth C. Healthcare groups at work: Further lessons from research into large scale coordination. *Cognition, Technology, and Work.* 2007;9(3):127–130.

21. Weick K. *Making Sense of the Organization.* London: Blackwell, 2001.

22. Dekker S. *The Field Guide to Human Error Investigations.* Aldershot, UK: Ashgate, 2002.

23. Zeleny M. The law of requisite variety: Is it applicable to human systems? *Human Systems Management.* 1986;6(4):269–271.

24. Mudge G. Airline safety: Can we break the old CRM paradigm? *Transportation Law Journal.* 1998;25(2):231–243.

25. Helmreich R. On error management: Lessons learned from aviation. *BMJ.* 2000 Mar 18;320(7237):781–785.

26. Militello LG, et al. The role of cognitive systems engineering in the system engineering design process. *Systems Engineering.* 2010;13(3):261–273.

27. Wright A, et al. A description and functional taxonomy of rule-based decision support content at a large integrated delivery network. *J Am Med Inform Assoc.* 2007;14(4):489–496.

28. Wakefield DS, et al. A general evaluation framework for analyzing data from the electronic health record: Verbal orders as a case in point. *Jt Comm J Qual Patient Saf.* 2012;38(10)444–451.

29. Koppel R, et al. Health care information technology to the rescue. In Koppel R, Gordon S, editors: *First, Do Less Harm: Confronting the Inconvenient Problems of Patient Safety.* Ithaca, NY: Cornell University Press, 2012, 62–89.

Chapter Eleven

MEASUREMENT STRATEGIES

Robert C. Lloyd, PhD

THE CONTEXT FOR HEALTH CARE MEASUREMENT

During the past 25 years, measurement of health care processes and outcomes has been rapidly evolving and changing. Initially, the focus was primarily on collecting data and merely publishing summary statistics. Little was being done in the early and mid-1980s to make sense out of data and produce information for decision making. Austin helped clarify this important distinction as follows[1(p. 24)]:

> *Data* refers to the raw facts and figures which are collected as part of the normal functioning of the hospital. Information, on the other hand, is defined as data, which have been processed and analyzed in a formal, intelligent way, so that the results are directly useful to those involved in the operation and management of the hospital.

Irrespective of how an individual interacts with the health care system, most would agree that it is information that is the desired end product not just a table of raw data. Whether you work at the bedside or in the laboratory, prepare medications in the pharmacy, perform surgery, make home care visits, or serve as the CEO of a large integrated delivery system, measurement has definitely become a central part of your daily work.

As interest in health care measurement and data has grown, we have seen the emergence of a new term—transparency. As discussed in Chapter 1, *transparency* involves open and easy access to information. Since the early 1990s, there has been a rapidly increasing demand for greater transparency around comparative data. Patients, families, the media, and political leaders have all started to ask, and in some cases demand, greater availability of information about health care outcomes and results. The assumption is that if patients and their families as well as purchasers and insurers of health care are provided with full data on health care processes and outcomes, better decisions could be made. The argument has been that the provider community has not readily and openly shared performance data with those seeking health care services.

The analogy used by many has been that consumers interested in purchasing a new car can get on the Internet and in 10 minutes find out all they need to know about the car they are thinking of buying. They can even get a rating of the "best" cars and see how the make and model they are considering compares to a larger class of similar cars. Now imagine, on the other hand, that you need to have your hip replaced. How would you go about determining which is the "best" hospital or group of surgeons to select for this procedure? Would you be able to obtain data on the hip surgeons in your area? What are the surgeons' infection rates? How many procedures does each surgical group perform each year? What type of implant(s) do they use? Do they regularly use the World Health Organization (WHO) Surgical Safety Checklist[2] before the start of surgery? Are the surgical groups you are considering willing to be transparent with their numbers and results? Even if they are willing to share some of their data, these are probably nowhere near what you can obtain when deciding on which car to select.

Transparency of results, therefore, has become one of the major challenges for health care professionals. What data do you release? How much detail do you release? Would you release data on individual physicians? Do you release data to the public? To the staff? How do you measure the performance of an individual physician or hospital? How much data do you need to make informed decisions? What are the "best" measures to collect? Do all data need to be severity or risk adjusted?

Ultimately, these issues boil down to a rather simple question: Do you know your data and results better than anyone else? If you do not, then it will be entirely too late to start thinking about your quality measurement journey when you are told there is a reporter from the local newspaper waiting in your office to talk with you about your organization's infection rates. It turns out that she obtained data from the state data commission on your organization's infection rates and is claiming that you are in the bottom 10% of your comparative group. Do you have a road map to guide your quality measurement journey or do you hope that the local reporter or TV crew picks the hospital down the street to interview?

A clear understanding of the skills needed to build a strong measurement component within your organization will not only allow you to respond effectively to current demands for data but will also position you well for the increasing focus on measurement that is present in the current and emerging health care landscape.

THE QUALITY MEASUREMENT JOURNEY

Measuring quality is a journey, and like any journey there are various stops along the way. The following sections describe these stops. Figures 11-1 and 11-2, below, illustrate the concepts discussed.

Setting Aims

All good measurement should be directly connected to the organization's mission or aim. You can test this yourself the next time you are working with an improvement team. Ask the members of the team if anyone can articulate which of the organization's aims are being maximized by the team's efforts? You will usually get blank stares when you ask this question. Some brave soul might respond, "I have no idea. We were told by our boss to improve this process." If the

employees of an organization do not understand and appreciate how measurement connects their work to the organization's purpose and objectives then they will be going through the motions but never connect the dots. Aims help answer the question "Why are you measuring?"

Determining Concepts

Concepts stem from high-level aims. Yet the concepts do not represent measurement. They essentially help to set the boundaries and focus for measurement and data collection. For example, in Figure 11-2 the aim is to have freedom from harm. This is the type of statement you will find frequently in an organization's mission statement. From this aim emerges a variety of concepts that address different aspects of harm (such as no infections, no medication errors, or no wrong-site surgeries). In Figure 11-2 the concept is reducing patient falls. We have become more specific by saying that we want to reduce patient falls as a form of harm but this is still not measurement. Reducing patient falls is a desired end state. It is not until you move to identifying a specific way to measure patient falls that you can actually take the first steps in the quality measurement journey.

Selecting Measures

We now have a number of options to consider as we move into the specific steps along the quality measurement journey. The first one is to decide which measure to select out of all the potential measures. If we stick with patient falls as the concept, we might consider the following measures:

Figure 11-1. The Quality Measurement Journey

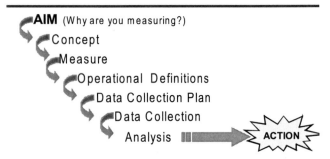

This figure illustrates the different stops along the quality measurement journey.

Source: R.C. Lloyd & Associates. Used with permission.

Figure 11-2. Examples of the Quality Measurement Journey

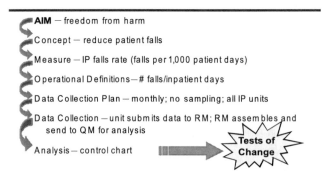

This figure provides examples for each stop along the journey.

Source: R.C. Lloyd & Associates. Used with permission.

A count. We could merely count the number of falls in a defined period of time, such as a day, a week, or a month. What does this give us? Is a count of the number of falls the most appropriate way to measure the concept of a patient fall? This month we had 26 falls. Last month we had 37. What does this tell us? It becomes even more challenging when you compare two hospitals. Hospitals A and B each had 35 falls this month. Which one is better? You don't know because you have no context for the number of falls. If I tell you, however, that Hospital A is a 530-bed urban teaching hospital, and Hospital B is a 210-bed community hospital, now you have context and would most likely say that it is not quite fair to compare the two hospitals because of differences in bed size, volume, location, and so on.

• *A percentage.* To compute the percentage of falls, we would need to define a denominator (for example, all inpatients who could possibly fall). The numerator would then be all the inpatients who fell once or more during their hospitalization and then aggregated for a defined period of time, such as a month or six months. With these two numbers, we could compute the percentage of patients who fell during the last month. Because a patient could fall more than once during his or her hospitalization, however, the percentage would not capture multiple falls.

A percentage is based on a binomial distribution. Measuring patient falls with a percentage, therefore, means that the team is not concerned with the specific number of times an individual patient fell but merely if the patient fell once or more. The question is simply, "Did this patient fall, yes or no?"

• *A rate.* This is the most frequently used measure to track the concept of patient falls. Like a percentage, a rate is still calculated by having a numerator and a denominator, but they are different from the ones we defined for a percentage. The numerator for a patient falls rate would be all patient falls, including multiples, during a defined period of time, such as a month. The denominator would then be the total number of patient-days in the month. This would produce an inpatient falls rate (for example, 3.2 falls per 1,000 patient-days).

Consider this example to help distinguish the differences between a percentage and a rate: A hospital with 210 discharges in a given month had a total of 47 of the 210 discharged patients fall once or more during their stay. From this information, you could conclude that 22.4% of the patients fell once or more (47 patient falls/210 patients = 22.4%. This is a straight percentage because you know only the percentage of patients who fell once or more, and multiple falls are ignored. Now, imagine that during the same month the actual total number of falls, including multiples, was 65, and the number of patient-days for the month equaled 5,621. When you divide the total number of falls by the total patient-days (65/5,621) you end up with .01156. Converting this ratio to a rate produces 11.56 falls per 1,000 patient-days. In this case, you have normalized the number of falls to a common denominator.

A percentage has the same type of unit in the numerator and denominator. In our previous example, the unit was patients. The question is, out of all patients how many of them fell? The distinguishing characteristic is whether they fell or not. In a rate calculation, you have two different types of units being compared. In our example, the two units were falls and patient-days. When you have two different types of units being used you cannot calculate a percentage.

Examples of potential measures for a variety of health care concepts can be found in Lloyd[3] (pages 69–71).

Defining Measures

After we have selected the specific measures we want to apply to our improvement project, we then need to be very clear about the operational definition of each measure. According to Deming, "An operational definition puts communicable meaning into a concept. Adjectives like good, reliable, uniform, round, tired, safe, unsafe, unemployed have no communicable meaning until they are expressed in operational terms of sampling, test, and criterion. The concept of a definition is ineffable: It cannot be communicated to someone else. An operational definition is one that reasonable men can agree on."[4(pp. 276–277)]

Stated a little differently, an operational definition is a description, in quantifiable terms, of what to measure and the specific steps needed to measure it consistently. A good operational definition does the following:

• Gives communicable meaning to a concept or idea
• Is clear and unambiguous
• Specifies the measurement method, procedures, and equipment (when appropriate)
• Provides decision-making criteria when necessary
• Enables consistency in data collection

Again, using the concept of a patient fall, it is necessary to ask, "What is the operational definition of a fall?" All falls are not the same. There are partial falls, near falls, falls with injuries, falls without an injury, and assisted falls. What is the difference between a partial fall and an assisted fall? Do we all agree on the characteristics of each one? If you sent out three people to collect data on partial falls would they all define a partial fall in the same way? Would the data be valid and reliable? Could you combine the data from the three people and have confidence that you were comparing apples to apples? If our operational definition of a partial fall was clear and unambiguous, and the people collecting the data all agreed that the defined criteria were reasonable, then they could proceed to collect data using a consistent operational definition. If the three people did not use consistent operational definitions, however, then you end up with fruit salad rather than apples compared to apples.

Additional detail on the critical role of operational definitions, as well as examples, can be found in Lloyd[3] (pages 71–75) and Provost and Murray[5] (pages 37–40).

Developing a Data Collection Plan and Collecting Data

After reaching consensus on the operational definitions for your measures, the next step in the quality measurement journey (*see* Figures 11-1 and 11-2) is to develop a data collection plan and then go out and actually gather the data. These two steps frequently run into roadblocks because team members or facilitators are not well versed in the methods and tools of data collection. A well-designed data collection strategy should address the following questions[6]:

- What process(es) will be monitored?
- What specific measures will be collected?
- What are the operational definitions of the measures?
- Why are you collecting these data? What is the rationale for collecting these data rather than other types of data?
- Will the data add value to your quality improvement efforts?
- Have you discussed the effects of stratification on the measures? (*See* below for more information on stratification.)
- How often (frequency) and for how long (duration) will you collect the data?
- Will you use sampling? If so, what sampling design have you chosen? (More information on sampling can be found in the section beginning on page 119.)

- How will you collect the data? What methods will you use? Possible methods include data sheets, surveys, focus group discussions, phone interviews, or some combination of these methods.
- Will you conduct a pilot study before you collect data for the entire organization?
- Who will collect the data? This is a critical question and, unfortunately, most improvement teams ignore it.
- What costs (monetary and time) will be incurred by collecting these data?
- Will collecting these data have negative effects on patients or employees?
- Do your data collection efforts need to be taken to your organization's institutional review board for approval?
- What are the current baseline measures?
- Do you have targets and goals for the measures?
- How will the data be coded, edited, and verified?
- Will you tabulate and analyze these data by hand or by computer?
- Are there confidentiality issues related to the use of the results?
- How will these data be used to make a difference?
- What plan do you have for disseminating the results of your data collection efforts?

Before beginning to collect data, team members must have a serious dialogue about these questions. In addition, team members must be familiar with and able to use the following key skills:

- Stratification
- Sampling

Stratification. This is the separation and classification of data into reasonably homogeneous categories. The objective of stratification is to create groupings that are reasonably homogeneous and as mutually exclusive as possible. Stratification is also used to uncover patterns that may be suppressed when all of the data are aggregated. Stratification allows understanding of differences in the data that might be due to the following:

- Day of the week (Mondays are very different from Wednesdays)
- Time of day (turnaround time is longer between 9 A.M. and 10 A.M. than it is between 3 P.M. and 4 P.M.)
- Time of year (we treat more flu patients in January than June)
- Shift (the process is different during day shift than during night shift)

- Type of order (stat versus routine)
- Type of procedure (nuclear medicine films versus routine x-rays)
- Type of machine (such as ventilators versus lab equipment)
- Patient characteristics that you believe have differential impacts on the selected outcome (for example, age, gender, prior admissions, or comorbid conditions)

Stratification is more of a logical issue than a statistical issue. It requires talking with people who have subject matter expertise, knowing how the process works, and identifying where pockets of variation may exist.

If your organization is planning to collect data on the culture of patient safety, for example, you should consider stratification. At some point you will most likely want to see the aggregated results for the entire organization. But the real value of improving the culture for patient safety comes with the ability to stratify the results by unit or employee categories (such as nurses, physicians, laboratory personnel, pharmacy personnel, or administration). It might also be very insightful to see if the culture scores differ by tenure with the organization, age of the employee, or the shift on which he or she works.

The objective of stratification is to drill down into the data to lend clarity to your analysis. The critical point for successful stratification is that you think about the stratification levels or categories *before* you actually embark on gathering the data. Once the data have been collected it is frequently too late or too time consuming to tease apart the stratification questions that may arise.

Further details on and examples of stratification can be found in Lloyd[3] (pages 75–79) and Provost and Murray[5] (pages 49–51).

Sampling. This is the second key skill needed during the data collection stage of your journey. Realize first of all that not every measure requires sampling. Sometimes there are small amounts of data, and sampling is not required or desirable. At other times you have ample data but the measure does not require that a subset of data be pulled from the total population. For example, if you want to know what percentage of patients receive appropriate medication reconciliation at time of discharge, you would most likely take all the patients discharged during the week or month (the denominator) and ask, "How many of these patient received appropriate medication reconciliation?" (the numerator). In this case, sampling

may not be necessary. However, when there is a fairly large amount of data and you cannot afford to spend the time or money to capture every occurrence of data, then sampling is appropriate. The question is, how do you draw your samples?

All too often health care professionals are not well-versed in sampling methods. As a result, they end up collecting too much data, too little data, or selecting data that do not adequately reflect the population they are trying to measure.

There are two basic approaches to sampling: *probability* and *nonprobability*. The dominant sampling techniques associated with each approach are shown below. The details on the advantages and disadvantages of the various sampling approaches can be found in Lloyd[3] (pages 79–94) and Provost and Murray[5] (pages 42–45). Practical discussions of sampling methods can be found in any basic text on statistical methods or research design.

Probability Sampling. Probability sampling methods are based on a simple principle: Within a known population of size n, there will be a fixed probability of selecting any single element (n_i). The selection of this element (and subsequent elements) must be determined by objective statistical means if the process is to be truly random (not affected by judgment, purposeful intent, or convenience). There are four basic approaches to probability sampling:

- *Systematic sampling* is achieved by numbering or ordering each element in the population—such as time order, alphabetical order, or medical record order—and then selecting every kth (k being a predetermined number) element. The key point that most people ignore when pulling a systematic sample is that the starting point for selecting every kth element should be generated through a random process. This approach has also been referred to as mechanical sampling.

- *Simple random sampling* is accomplished by giving every element in the population an equal and independent chance of being included in the sample. A random number generator or a random number table is usually used to devise a random selection process.

- *Stratified random sampling* results when stratification is applied to a population and then a random process is used to pull samples from within each stratum. This approach helps ensure that different groups within the population have a chance (probability) of being selected, which may not be the case with a simple random sample.

• *Stratified proportional random sampling* is a little more complex because it requires figuring out what proportion each stratum represents in the total population then replicating this proportion in the sample that is randomly pulled from each stratum. To successfully use this approach as well as stratified random sampling, you need to have sufficiently large populations so that you can divide them into smaller stratification levels and still have enough data from which to draw an appropriate sample. For example, if you stratify by gender, age, race, and prior hospitalization within the last 30 days, you may wind up with a category—such as black females older than 65 years of age who were in the hospital within the last 30 days—that contains only 6 patients. In this case, you have stratified by so many levels that you have reduced the number of patients to a point that sampling does not make sense.

Nonprobability Sampling. Nonprobability sampling methods are usually used when the researcher is not interested in being able to generalize the findings to a larger population. The basic objective of nonprobability sampling is to select a sample that the researchers believe is "typical" of the larger population. A chief criticism of these approaches to sampling is that there is no way to factually measure if the nonprobability sample is representative of the population from which it is drawn. Samples pulled this way are assumed to be "good enough" for the people drawing the sample but the findings should not be generalized to larger populations.

• *Convenience sampling* is the classic "man on the street" interview approach to sampling. In this case, a reporter may select four or five people standing on the train platform (who look interesting or approachable) and ask them what they think of the local school referendum. While these interviews may provide interesting sound bites, they should not be used to arrive at a conclusion that "this is how the people feel on this issue."

Convenience sampling typically contains considerable bias (usually the biases of the individual collecting the data). For example, if you want to gather feedback from patients in the emergency department (ED) and you tell a staff person to "go talk to a few people about their experience in the ED" you could very well end up with a biased convenience sample. The staff person will most likely not select a person to interview who looks upset or bothered, but instead select the kind-looking elderly woman who is waiting for her daughter to receive a few stitches for a nonserious cut on her

hand. She is more than happy to talk to someone while waiting for her daughter's discharge. This selection bias in the sampling plan can produce results that are certainly convenient but not very generalizable.

• *Quota sampling* is frequently used with convenience sampling. When this is done, the staff person referenced above knows that she needs to get a total of 10 respondents (the quota). So she is focused on getting these 10 interviews; not 8 and not 11, but a quota of 10. This is done frequently in health care when a quota of 10 charts or 8 patient interviews is set as the desired amount of data. There are steps that can be taken in developing quota samples[7] to ensure reasonably robust data. Unfortunately, most of the time these steps are not followed, and the quota sample represents a fairly weak approach to sampling.

• *Judgment sampling* is frequently used in quality improvement initiatives. Judgment sampling relies on the knowledge of subject matter experts. These individuals can tell you when the performance of a process varies and when this variation should be observed. For example, if the admitting clerk tells you that patients "bunch up" between 0830 and 0930 and that this is a very different situation than what she observes between 1500 and 1600, then you should consider sampling differently during these two time periods. Similarly, if a staff nurse tells you that "things get crazy around here at 1100 due to discharge timing," then you would want to create a sampling plan for "crazy time" and "non-crazy time." The critical point for judgment sampling is that the person offering the judgment needs to be credible and respected by those working in the process. Otherwise, bias increases dramatically in this form of sampling.

Building knowledge of sampling methods is one of the best things you can do to enhance your data collection processes. Good sampling techniques help to ensure the validity and reliability of the data you will take to the next step in your quality improvement journey—analysis.

Analyzing Data

Figure 11-3 on page 121 depicts the process by which data are turned into information. Central to this process is the analytic step (the "Data Analysis and Output" box at the bottom of the figure). Notice that the analysis of data must be placed in the appropriate context. Otherwise it is an exercise with no real purpose. Also remember that data collection and statistical analysis of the data are not the objectives. Data and their analysis provide a springboard for the real objectives—learning and improvement.

The analytical and interpretive steps the team must apply to the data are critical to any successful improvement project. Frequently, however, teams fail to engage in planning for the analysis of the data they collect, which causes them to hit yet another roadblock. To be successful at this point in your journey, you need to think about the following questions:

• Who will be responsible for organizing the data after they are collected?

• If the data have been manually collected who will be responsible for assembling all the data collection forms?

• Did you remember to place a unique identification number on each chart, survey, or log sheet?

• If appropriate, have you set up a codebook for the data?

• How will you enter the data into the computer? Will you scan the data into a computer, enter them manually, or create an automatic download from an existing database?

• Who will enter the data? Will you verify the data after they have been entered? If you have a large volume of data—like the volume generated by surveys—have you con-

sidered using a professional data entry service?

• Who will be responsible for analyzing the data? (This question applies whether you are performing manual or automated analysis.)

• What computer software will you use? Will you produce descriptive statistical summaries, cross-tabulations, graphic summaries, or control charts?

• Do you have control charting software?

• After you have analyzed the data, who will be responsible for translating the raw numbers into information for decision making?

• Will you need to develop a written summary of the results? If so, who will be given this responsibility?

• Are there different audiences that need to receive the results and have they requested different report formats?

Probably the greatest challenge a quality improvement team will face at this step is whether they will approach the analysis of data from a static or dynamic point of view. Most health care professionals have received statistical training that is grounded in static or enumerative approaches to data. Static approaches to data analysis are designed to compare the results from the first time period (for example, the medication error rate last month) with the results at the second

Figure 11-3. The Process of Turning Data into Information for Decision Making

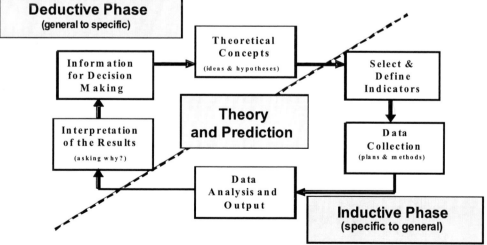

This figure illustrates how your organization can move from data to information for decision making.

Source: Adapted from Lloyd, R.: *Quality Health Care: A Guide to Developing and Using Indicators.* Sudbury, MA: Jones and Bartlett Publishers, 2004. Used with permission.

time period (this month) and raise the question– are the two numbers different? Research conducted in this manner is referred to as *static group comparisons.*[8]

It is a pretty well-established fact that if you compare two numbers, there is a fairly high likelihood that one number will be different from the other. Some analysts and managers will apply the "interocular test of significance" and conclude that the two numbers certainly look different. If you want to be a little more precise, however, you will apply statistical tests of significance to see if the two data points are statistically different at the .01 or .05 level of significance.

Figure 11-4, at right, provides an example of a static display of data. In this example, we are looking at the percentage mortality associated with doing coronary artery bypass surgery (CABG) before and after a new protocol is put in place. Note that the larger block on the left side of the diagram reflects a 5% mortality, while the smaller block on the right depicts a mortality of 4%. Some people might get quite excited about the decrease from 5% to 4% and even claim that it is a "significant drop in mortality." Others might point out that it represents a 20% decrease in mortality. Still others might choose to merely look at the size of the big block on the left and the relatively small size of the block on the right and conclude that things have improved. Although this chart may look impressive, the issue is not the size of the blocks or even the average percentage mortality. From a quality improvement perspective, the key question is, "What is the variation in the CABG mortality at Time 1 compared to Time 2?"

Static group comparisons, although popular in health care, are not the preferred approach when conducting quality improvement research. The best analytic path to follow for measurement of quality and safety, therefore, is one guided by statistical process control methods (SPC). This branch of statistics was developed initially by Walter A. Shewhart in the early 1920s while he worked at Western Electric Company.[9] It focuses primarily on analyzing the inherent variation that lives in data and doing so by plotting data over time not by using aggregated data and summary statistics, such as the average and standard deviation, to make conclusions about the data. Aggregated data presented in tabular formats or with summary statistics will not help you understand the variation in the process or measure the impact of process improvement efforts.

Figure 11-4. A Static Display of Data

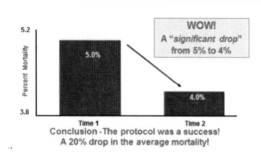

This figure shows an example of one way to display data that may overstate success because it only compares averages.

Source: R.C. Lloyd & Associates. Used with permission.

Variation exists in all processes. Consider your morning commute to work. If you ask people how long it takes to get to work, they usually reply, "Oh about X number of minutes." Unless you live across the street from where you work, there will always be variation in your commute time. It never takes precisely the same amount of time each day. There is normal variation (for example, between 35 and 55 minutes each day), and then there are times when a special event, such as an accident or bad weather, knocks you out of your regular commuting pattern and makes your commute significantly longer than normal.

The best way to understand the variation that lives in your data, therefore, is to plot the data over time. Let's return to our example of CABG mortality to see what this measure actually represents. In Figure 11-5 on page 123, we see that the data found in Figure 11-4 are plotted over time on a control chart. This offers a very different view of the data than we observed previously. We notice that the mortality started quite high (about 9%) and decreased continuously until it reached approximately 2%, where it stayed for about three months. But we also notice that after the protocol was introduced, the mortality actually started to climb until now where it hovers around 7%. Yet the first average remains 5%, while the second average remains 4%. How is it that the average could drop but the process is actually producing higher percentages of mortality? The reason is due to the manner in which an average is calculated. It merely adds up all the numbers and divides by the total number of data points. The average is not designed to represent the variation in the process over time. In fact, time is stripped away from the data when we compute an average or any other descriptive statistic. The issue here is that the static view (the average) can be very misleading if you do not understand the underlying variation in the process.

The use of run and control charts allows an improvement team to analyze data as a continuous stream that has a rhythm and pattern. Statistical tests are used to detect whether the process performance reflects what Shewhart classified as *common cause variation* or *special cause variation*. Decisions about improvement strategies and their impacts will be based on understanding the type of variation that lives in the process, not on whether one data point is different from another.[3,5,8,10–15]

Taking Action

The final step in the quality measurement journey involves taking *action* to make improvements. All the preceding steps are designed to lead to this milestone in the journey. Data without a context or plan for action give the team a false sense of accomplishment. It is not until you identify change concepts and specific ideas that you believe will move process performance in the desired direction, and conduct

Figure 11-5. A Static Display of Data

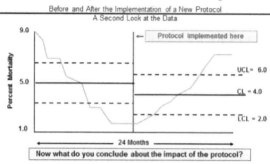

This figure shows a way to plot data over time. The data found here are the same as those shown in Figure 11-4; however, the presentation paints a much different picture of performance.

Source: R.C. Lloyd & Associates. Used with permission.

tests of change (*see* Chapter 12, pages 126–127), that the journey is complete. All too often, however, health care managers and leaders see data as the beginning and end of the journey. The data merely allow us to set the direction of our improvement journey, not define where the journey will take us.

REFERENCES

1. Austin CJ. *Information Systems for Hospital Administration,* 2nd ed. Chicago: Health Administration Press, 1983.
2. World Health Organization (WHO). *WHO Guidelines for Safe Surgery 2009: Safe Surgery Saves Lives.* Geneva: WHO, 2009. Accessed Nov 1, 2012. http://www.who.int/patientsafety/safesurgery/tools_resources/9789241598552/en/.
3. Lloyd R. *Quality Health Care: A Guide to Developing and Using Indicators.* Sudbury, MA: Jones and Bartlett, 2004.
4. Deming W. *Out of the Crisis.* 1982. Cambridge, MA: MIT Press, 2000.
5. Provost LP, Murray SK. *The Health Care Data Guide: Learning from Data for Improvement.* San Francisco: Jossey-Bass, 2011.
6. Lloyd RC. The search for a few good indicators. In Ransom SB, Joshi MS, Nash DB, editors: *The Healthcare Quality Book: Vision, Strategy, and Tools.* Chicago: Health Administration Press, 2005, 89–116.
7. Babbie ER. *The Practice of Social Research.* Belmont, CA: Wadsworth, 1979.
8. Benneyan JC, Lloyd RC, Plsek PE. Statistical process control as a tool for research and health care improvement. *Qual Saf Health Care.* 2003;12(6):458–464.
9. Schultz LE. *Profiles in Quality: Learning from the Masters.* New York City: Quality Resources, 1994.
10. Carey RG. *Improving Healthcare with Control Charts: Basic and Advanced SPC Methods and Case Studies.* Milwaukee: ASQ Quality Press, 2003.
11. Carey RG, Lloyd RC. *Measuring Quality Improvement in Healthcare: A Guide to Statistical Process Control Applications.* Milwaukee: ASQ Quality Press, 2001.
12. Western Electric Co. *Statistical Quality Control Handbook.* Indianapolis: AT&T Technologies, 1985.
13. Mohammed MA, Worthington P, Woodall WH. Plotting basic control charts: Tutorial notes for healthcare practitioners. *Qual Safety Health Care.* 2008;17(2)137–145.
14. Wheeler DJ. *Advanced Topics in Statistical Process Control: The Power of Shewhart's Charts.* Knoxville, TN: SPC Press, 1995.
15. Wheeler DJ, Chambers DS. *Understanding Statistical Process Control.* Knoxville, TN: SPC Press, 1992.

Chapter Twelve

CARE PROCESS
IMPROVEMENT

Allan Frankel, MD; Carol Haraden, PhD; David Munch, MD

Standardizing procedures, introducing structured communication techniques, implementing WalkRounds (*see* Chapter 5), redesigning patient education materials, deploying a computerized provider order entry system. What do all these actions have in common? They all involve improvement. Taking what was and making it better. Putting in the new to replace or enhance the old. Although it is easy to say we must improve our processes, without a systematic approach to doing that, such efforts can and probably will fail. At the very least they will not go as smoothly as they should, and the resulting processes will not be as good as they could be.

There are many different ways to structure the improvement process; far too many, in fact, to be covered completely by this book. However, the following sections of this chapter address some common methods that have been used successfully across many types of health care organizations within many different types of processes.

THE MODEL FOR IMPROVEMENT

The Model for Improvement is a straightforward effective tool for accelerating change.[1] The model has two main parts:

1. The following three fundamental questions, which organizations must address for each process being improved:

  a. What are we trying to accomplish?

  b. How will we know that change is an improvement?

  c. What changes can we make that will result in improvement?

2. The Plan-Do-Study-Act (PDSA) cycle to test and implement changes: The PDSA cycle guides the change process and helps determine if a change results in an improvement.[2]

To answer the previous questions and drive improvement forward, you must engage in the following activities:

• Establish a team. Including the right people on a process improvement team is critical to a successful effort. Although teams can vary in size and composition, they should include individuals familiar with all the different parts of the process to be improved, including physicians, pharmacists, nurses, and other frontline workers, as well as managers and administrators. The team must include individuals representing three different kinds of expertise within your organization: system leadership, technical expertise, and day-to-day leadership. Without these different kinds of input, improvement will not move forward effectively.

A system leader has enough authority in your organization to institute a change that has been suggested and overcome barriers that arise. He or she has the authority to allocate the time and resources for the project and understands both the implications of a proposed change for various parts of the system and the more remote consequences that a change might trigger.

A clinical technical expert is someone who knows the subject being addressed intimately and understands the processes of care associated with that subject. An expert on improvement methods can provide additional technical support to a performance improvement team by helping the team determine what to measure, assisting in design of simple, effective measurement tools, and providing guidance on collection, interpretation, and display of data.

A day-to-day leader is the driver of the project, ensuring that tests are implemented and overseeing data collection. It is important that this person understands not only the details of the system under study, but also the various effects of making change(s) in the system.

• Clearly state the goals or aims of the performance improvement project. A project aim should be specific, numerical, and measurable. It should describe the system to be improved and the patient population affected by the improvement, and it should be tied into the organization's strategic goals and values. It should set a time line for achievement and communicate that maintaining the status quo is not an option. Setting such aims helps to create tension for change, directs measurement, and focuses initial changes. An example of a well-defined aim might be to "reduce adverse events in the ICU by 75% within 11 months" or "achieve 100% compliance with the Universal Protocol for Preventing Wrong Site, Wrong Procedure, Wrong Person Surgery™[3] within the next six months." Team members must agree on the aims of a project and be careful not to deliberately back away or "drift" away from an aim unconsciously. Regular repetition of the aim can help prevent this.

• Establish measures. As discussed in Chapter 11, by developing specific measures, creating a data collection plan, and collecting data to measure the success in meeting identified aims, organizations can determine whether an initiative actually leads to an improvement.

• Identify changes that are most likely to result in improvement. While not all changes lead to improvement, all improvement requires change. Changes that work in your environment will most likely stem from some general approaches or concepts that have worked in other organizations. While there are literally hundreds of change concepts from which you can develop specific changes, following is a brief list of some of the more common concepts:

—Eliminate waste. This involves systematically looking for ways of eliminating any activity or resource in your organization that does not add value. A critical tool in eliminating waste is Lean Methodology. (See a further discussion of Lean Methodology on pages 128–133.)

—Improve work flow.

—Optimize inventory. This ties in neatly with reducing waste, as inventory of all types is a possible source of waste in organizations.

—Change the work environment. This could include both the physical environment and the cultural environment.

—Improve your relationship with patients.

—Manage time. This may include wait times, turnover times, or lead times. For example, organizations may focus on changes that decrease delays in the emergency department (ED) waiting room, improve the turnover times of operating rooms, or decrease the lead times necessary for critical tests.

—Reduce variation. As discussed in Chapter 4, reducing variation—also known as standardization—improves the predictability of outcomes and helps reduce the frequency of poor results.

—Increase reliability. Organizations can reduce errors by redesigning processes to make it less likely for people to make errors. This may involve implementing checklists, closed-loop communication cycles, or other such tools.

• Test changes on a small scale. After generating change ideas, test a change or group of changes on a small scale to see if they result in improvement. *Small scale* means such tests may involve 1 individual or 10 individuals, but invariably involve a smaller number than suggested by clinicians with limited improvement expertise. Small tests of change are never successes or failures, they are simply an opportunity for learning. There are many reasons to test changes, including the following:

—Tests verify that a change will result in improvement.

—Tests predict how much improvement can be expected from a change.

—Tests identify areas for improvement that can be quickly addressed on a more reasonable scale.

—Tests can help minimize resistance upon full implementation of a change.

—When beginning to test changes, you should pick easy changes to try. Look for the concepts that seem most feasible and will have the greatest impact.

—Teams should test changes using the Plan-Do-Study-Act model.[2] First developed by Walter A. Shewhart as the Plan-Do-Check-Act (PDCA) cycle, the system was modified by W. Edwards Deming who changed Shewhart's cycle to PDSA, replacing "Check" with "Study."[4] Within the model there are four main steps.

—Step 1: Plan. This step involves planning for the test of change. Within this step teams should answer the following questions:

○ What is the objective of the test?

○ What do we predict will happen during the test and why?

○ How will we perform the test?

○ Who will be involved? It's best to start the first PDSA cycle with willing participants. Some individuals are more enthusiastic to work with new ideas than others. Rogers, who calls these individuals early adopters and innovators, reports that they enjoy the experience of tweaking a process or idea until it works in their environment. On the flip side, late adopters are individuals who throw up roadblocks or downright refuse to try a new process or approach unless they are certain that all the potential pitfalls, complications, and problems with the process have been addressed.[5] When testing a change, you should work with the early adopters first and then work through the rest of the population, ultimately introducing the process to the late adopters.

○ When will we perform the test?

○ Where will we perform the test?

○ How will we measure success? What measures will we use and how will we collect data?

—Step 2: Do. This step involves carrying out the test on a small scale. During the "Do" step, team members should document problems and unexpected observations and begin to analyze the data

—Step 3: Study. As discussed in Chapter 11, data analysis is critical to any improvement project. Team members should set aside time to review data, see how they compare to the predictions, and summarize what was learned. Teams should reflect on the results of every change. After making a change, a team should ask: What did we expect to happen? What did happen? Were there unintended consequences? What was the best thing about this change? the worst? What might we do next? Too often, people avoid reflecting on failure. Remember that teams often learn very important lessons from tests of change that don't achieve what is predicted.

—Step 4: Act. On the basis of the results of the previous step, the Act step involves refining the change and preparing for the next test. If the test shows that a change is not leading to improvement, that knowledge is important too. "Failed" tests of change are a natural part of the improvement process; they indicate a direction to not go. If a team experiences very few failed tests of change, it is probably not pushing the boundaries of innovation very far.

Small tests of change are just that—small. It is better to conduct more PDSA cycles of small changes than fewer cycles of bigger changes. *Consider the following example of how one team used PDSA to test a small change: A 250-bed community hospital was working on a program to implement planned patient visits for blood sugar management. To test the change on a small scale, the organization worked with a physician who was excited about the program and willing to participate in the change process. She implemented the following PDSA test:*

Plan: Ask one patient if he or she would like more information on how to manage his or her blood sugar.

Do: Dr. J asked her first patient with diabetes on Tuesday.

Study: Patient was interested; Dr. J was pleased at the positive response.

Act: Dr. J will continue with the next five patients and set up a planned visit for those who say "yes."

The tempo with which the repeating tests of change occurs will determine the speed with which the actual process becomes more reliable. Testing every day or every other day results in a key process improvement every couple of weeks. Testing once a week results in key process improvement every three to four months. The speed of testing is the key to the speed of implementation and spread.

• Implement changes. After testing a change on a small scale, learning from each test, and refining the change through several PDSA cycles, the team can implement the change on a broader scale—for example, for an entire pilot population or on an entire unit. During implementation, teams learn valuable lessons necessary for successful spread, including key infrastructure issues, optimal sequencing of tasks, and working with people to help them adopt and adapt to a change.

• Spread the changes. After successful implementation of a change for a pilot population or an entire unit, the team can spread the changes to other parts of the organization or to other organizations. For example, if all 30 nurses on a pilot unit successfully implement a new medication reconciliation and order form, then *spread* would be replicating this change sequentially in all nursing units in the organization and assisting the units in adopting or adapting to the change.

By using the Model for Improvement to drive improvement, organizations can quickly implement changes that achieve measurable results. As long as team members have change ideas to try, this model is effective at testing and implementing to achieve success.

LEAN METHODOLOGY

Toyota Production System or "Lean" production is an effective method for advancing patient safety that achieves reliability by developing processes that reduce or prevent errors, mitigate errors if they do occur, and engage frontline staff in continuous improvement. Lean focuses on process flow, visual management, creation of standard work, development of staff skills in problem identification and resolution, and responsiveness to defects or errors.

Lean is not only a tool for process improvement but an organizational approach to reliability based on a set of explicit guiding principles that guide staff to provide defect-free and safe care.[6] It involves leadership and management systems that continuously coach and develop staff to continuously surface problems and solve them. Although often used to improve clinical processes and systems, this philosophy and these tools are equally applicable in "soft process" areas, such as new product development, employee orientation, accounting/finance, and customer service.

Lean supports two different performance improvement methodologies: A3 and Rapid Improvement Events (RIEs).[7] A3 is used for smaller-scale issues that arise on a daily basis, while RIEs are used for more complex processes. Similar steps are found in both approaches. The problem or current process is thoroughly evaluated before countermeasures for improvement are entertained. Both approaches build in project management for successful implementation, and both create learning.

Using A3 Methodology

A foundational element of Lean is the daily management of problems. As discussed throughout this book, hospitals and health systems are complex, and problems arise on a daily basis. "Work-arounds" allow the problems to surface again and again, contributing to the chaos and risk in the work environment. Effective problem solving requires identifying issues as quickly as possible and responding immediately such that the problem can be mitigated before harm can come to the patient.

Surfacing problems quickly requires visual and daily management systems, which may entail visual signals that something is wrong, regular observation of work to identify problems, timely measurement systems that record performance at the process level, and responsiveness when errors occur. As mentioned earlier, error response needs to be one of coaching and support that advances a safe culture and educates the caregiver, not a punitive action.

A3 is a methodology for solving small-scope problems or responding to incidents that arise on a daily basis. It uncovers and addresses the root cause of an issue, which is critically important, so that the problem does not return. (*A3* refers to the size of the paper [11-inch by 17-inch] on which A3 reports are usually recorded. The issue, problem, and cause are recorded on the left side; the countermeasure, project plan, metrics, and reflection are recorded on the right side.)

A3 problem solving starts with stating the issue. The problem is then investigated thoroughly by a team. Questions the team may want to ask include the following:
- What happened?
- How often does this occur?
- What are the upstream and downstream influences?
- How long has this been occurring?
- What are the results of the interviews with staff from that area?
- How difficult will the problem be to solve?

Graphical representation of the problem is encouraged, as opposed to a narrative approach. After the problem has been investigated thoroughly, the team can then determine the cause. There are many tools you can use to help determine the cause, including cause-and-effect diagrams and the 5-Whys tool. The 5-Whys tool involves asking "why" enough times to get to the root cause.

After the team determines the root cause, it can propose countermeasures that address the problem. The team puts a plan in place to implement the countermeasures. This plan should address the who, what, when, where, and how of implementation and define follow-up measures to determine if the countermeasures have been effective.

Critical to the A3 process are conversations among stakeholders that build consensus and agreement around problem analysis and the countermeasures. When agreement is reached, the likelihood of success is much higher.

A sample A3 is shown in Figure 12-1 (page 129).

Rapid Improvement Event (RIE)

When using Lean Methodology to improve complex processes, your organization must first start with a high-level analysis of the particular service line or department being examined from a customer value perspective—the customer

Figure 12-1. Respiratory Therapy A3

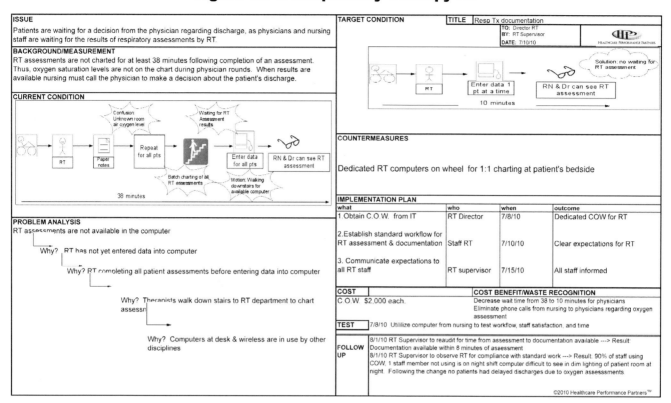

This figure presents a sample A3, which was performed to improve a barrier to patient discharge—timely charting by the respiratory therapist. RT, respiratory therapy; Tx, treatment; COW, computer on wheels; IT, information technology.

Source: David Munch. © 2010 Healthcare Performance Partners.SM Used with permission.

being the patient. The patient's journey through the clinical process is mapped step-by-step from beginning to end. This sequence of process steps, which is intended to provide value to the patient, is called the Value Stream and is recorded in the Value Stream Map. The map is then analyzed, and the sequence of processes is segregated into process groups or "chunks" that can now be improved through a series of "Rapid Improvement Events" (RIEs). (*See* Sidebar 12-1 on page 130 for some examples of processes that were improved using Lean.)

An RIE is a two- to five-day event in which a process or a component of a process is analyzed and improved through the work of an integrated team. The RIE serves several purposes:

1. To improve and standardize a particular process, reduce waste, and improve reliability using Lean principles

2. To grow the team's knowledge of Lean methods and problem-solving skills through just-in-time training and the experience of the RIE

3. To establish a culture of continuous improvement. Over the course of time, with multiple RIEs involving multiple members of the service line, cultural change takes place. Adherence to standard work and the skills for improvement become values and practices that are strengthened. A learning organization evolves.

Steps Involved in a Rapid Improvement Event

There are several steps involved in an RIE. Different organizations can take various approaches to these steps. The following sections take a brief look at one way to approach them.

Preparation. Preparation for RIEs starts with a planning phase in which leaders select improvement team members and prepare the team members for the event. Team members establish baseline measures, solicit input from members of the service line, schedule the improvement event, and determine implementation time lines.

The majority of the RIE team members come from the front line because they are the people who do the work. They have the most in-depth understanding of the current work and the most knowledge of the opportunities for improvement. Their contribution on the team provides for greater improvement and comes with credibility that cannot be achieved with a top-down approach. Because of their participation, it is much more likely that sustained improvement will be realized.

Each RIE team has a lead, a facilitator, and an executive champion assigned to support the work. The lead's major responsibility is to manage the project to completion. The facilitator is skilled in facilitation methods and serves to guide the process of the RIE and ensure that all members participate. The executive champion participates on the team and supports the team's work, addressing barriers if they occur.

Sidebar 12-1. Examples of Lean Improved Processes

Example: Our pharmacy evaluated the medication ordering process and found 142 steps in the current state. The future state had only 100 steps arranged in a much more efficient order with less chance of error.

Example: Pharmacists were spending an inordinate amount of time searching for lab values in the lab data system for their assessments of medication orders. The computers were programmed to automatically bring the information to the screen, doubling the efficiency of the pharmacist in the order review process.

Example: Shift change between nurses was observed. The receiving nurse was relying on the verbal report and the patient information found in the electronic record. The off-shift written nursing summary was not being used because it was redundant, yet had been "tradition." This portion of the handoff process was stopped altogether, saving significant time in duplicate documentation.

Example: Chemotherapy infusion orders were evaluated for adjustments for weight and kidney function, and gaps were observed. Protocols and forcing functions were implemented to ensure first-time quality.

Source: David Munch. Used with permission.

Step 1: The current-state analysis is performed. At the beginning of the RIE, the agenda for the event is reviewed, team-building exercises take place, and norms are established. This is a good time to provide just-in-time teaching for the improvement team for approximately one hour with a review of Lean principles and tools. The RIE that follows imbeds Lean skills into the team thus providing experiential training.

When these activities are completed, the "current state" is analyzed. This is done by recording each step in a particular process on a whiteboard or on sticky notes and placing them on the wall. Each step is placed in order, and if there is variability of a particular step, the variations are stacked vertically on the first variation. Rework loops are drawn and the layout of the floor, movement patterns, material locations, and work patterns are evaluated. The process is evaluated for evidence of waste using the following categories:

- Overprocessing
- Waiting
- Excess inventory
- Excess movement of people
- Excess transport of materials
- Defects
- Overproduction of services or product
- Unused employee creativity

The learning proceeds and awareness grows. At the start, members of the team rarely have the same perception of the current process. The sharing of perceptions forces the realization of the previously unappreciated variability and brings the team to a common mental model of the current state.

This mapping process is not complete until the improvement team goes to where the work is performed and observes the process directly to see if the map they created in the classroom is an accurate representation of the work. It never is. Invariably, additions and revisions occur based on direct observation. Observing the process helps the team visually appreciate the profound variability and unnecessary complexity of the process in which they work. The waste becomes apparent.

Process and outcome measures of the current state are determined, and data are collected either before or during this step. Future measures are determined to track the effectiveness of the new process, the implementation plan, and the evidence that improvement is being sustained.

Step 2: The future state is developed. After they analyze the current state of the process and agree on a common mental model, the team evaluates each step in the process using the following criteria:

1. Does this step bring value to the customer?: "Value Add" "Non Value Add (NVA)"

2. If not, is it necessary?: "Non Value Necessary" "Non Value Unnecessary"

The ratio of value added to NVA steps is typically 1 to 10, a remarkably low number.

After evaluating all the steps, the team then proceeds to take away the NVA unnecessary steps, occasionally taking out whole groups of steps that can be done in a more efficient manner. Team members evaluate and redesign remaining processes, taking out waste using Lean methods to provide more effective work.

Teams hold "stakeholder" sessions at the end of steps 1 and 2 where the improvement team's colleagues from the service line get to review the work and provide input. This is a critical step to build ownership and buy-in from the larger clinical team.

Step 3: The test of change is performed and observed. After a process has been redesigned, the new process is tried on the unit under direct observation of the team members. Members from the unit get to participate in this test and provide input. The information and measures from this test are evaluated and are used to improve the future state of the process design.

Step 4: The new process is finalized, including implementation plan, metrics, time lines, and roles. The project plan is set in this step, starting with the implementation and communication plans. The team makes plans to observe the implementation on a regular basis, such as daily, weekly, monthly, and then quarterly. Assignments are made. Resources are aligned. Support departments are commonly brought in at this time. For example, the facilities team may need to move a piece of equipment, information technology may need to add a computer terminal, and data support may need to develop a report.

Step 5: The communication plan to stakeholders is developed. A "Celebration" is held where the executive team, directors, members from the involved service line, and other interested parties come to hear about the RIE activity, the new process that has been developed, the improvements that are expected, and the plans for implementation. Learning occurs here. Directors and others have the opportunity to evaluate the ideas for their areas, to understand their role in supporting this work, and to see that the organization is serious about improvement. This is one of the first opportunities for acknowledgment and validation in a meaningful way. Within this step, questions are asked and understanding grows. One of the more common questions asked of the team is: "What have you learned?"

Step 6: The new process is implemented. During this step, the team manages organizationwide implementation. Management plays a critical role in this phase and must be knowledgeable of the new work and able to coach the staff. Project management skills are critical here, and leadership support will be needed. The new standard process is observed daily for 2 to 4 weeks. If process control is achieved, the observations become less frequent over the course of 3 to 12 months. Coaching the staff to the new standard process occurs within this step.

The team must also be able to revise the standard process if an unanticipated issue surfaces that justifies a revision. It is critical here to improve and adhere to a standard process and not reach for a work-around.

It is also important to make the work as visible as possible, tracking the measures such that everyone can see them. Visual control boards and data walls are effective for making work visible. It is important to keep data simple and understandable. It may be helpful to use tally sheets, run charts, bar graphs, colors, and any method that identifies defects quickly such that response can be immediate.

Step 7: The plan for sustaining the work is developed. This is a critical phase requiring ongoing support and vigilance. Improvements that are not sustained are an enormous drain on human resources. All previous efforts that have gone into improving the process are wasted, and the culture of work-arounds is reinforced. Consequently, planning for an improvement event requires a plan to sustain the work.

There are many variables that determine sustainable success, including the strength of organization leadership, management, staff, organizational goals, clarity/alignment to the standard work, information management, and others. Some process designs will require more work to sustain than others. For example, if the work has forcing functions, there will be less need for vigilance because choice and opportunity to deviate from the standard are restricted. (More information about forcing functions can be found in

Chapter 4.) For other processes, it is important to set up systems such that deviations from the standard are recognized and responded to as quickly as possible. This can be done through visual management, timely measurement systems, and observation. There needs to be ongoing monitoring and measuring at the process level, and there needs to be a timely response when errors are encountered.

To effectively manage sustainability, managers will need to be supported with skill development and redeployment of their time. In this context, redeployment means looking at a manager's current work and relieving him or her of wasteful or unnecessary tasks so there is available time to do the work described above. If this is not done, these people who are already working very hard will find it difficult or impossible to perform the management functions required to sustain the standard work developed in the rapid improvement events.

The Four Rules of Process Improvement

There is a very effective construct for process design called "The Four Rules."[8] These rules can serve to guide the design, operation, and improvement of every process—whether you are using A3 or RIE. The rules are as follows:

Rule 1: All work shall be highly specified as to content, sequence, timing, and outcome. This provides a guide for the evaluation of current process and the creation of future standard work by addressing the following: What should be done, in what order, by what time, and the expectation for outcomes should be X. The more the work is specified, the easier it is to identify the error. You can't identify the abnormal until you specify the normal. In a variable environment, it is easy to assume an error is just another variation. Rule 1 provides a construct to create standard work such that error is obvious.

Rule 2: Every customer-supplier connection must be direct and there must be an unambiguous yes-or-no way to send requests and receive responses. There are many handoffs in health care. If they are not performed well, medical errors can occur. This rule provides a guide for reliable and safe handoffs and transitions.

Rule 3: The pathway for every product and service must be simple and direct. The more choice we have, the more likely we'll make the wrong choice. Simplifying and specifying the path of services as much as possible will reduce errors.

Rule 4: Any improvement must be made in accordance with the scientific method, under the guidance of a teacher, at the lowest possible level in the organization. Despite our best efforts, problems will arise. Those problems must be dealt with effectively such that harm does not find its way to the patient. Having a staff that is actively surfacing problems and solving them (through A3 and RIEs) is a critical element of patient safety.

The 14 Principles

Lean also offers 14 principles that can be used to guide the design of future state processes. Some of the more relevant principles for health care are as follows[6]:

(Principle 2) Create process "flow" to surface problems. Design the sequence of services to be given one at a time in a smooth order based on patient demand without waiting. Patient or provider waiting indicates a problem and points to the opportunity to improve work flow.

(Principle 4) Level out the workload (Heijunka). Variable workload overwhelms the staff and increases the likelihood of error. Design processes to match capacity with demand and level demand as much as possible.

(Principle 5) Stop when there is a quality problem (Jidoka). Design systems to recognize defects or errors immediately and respond immediately. An example of this in many hospitals is the rapid response team.

(Principle 6) Standardize tasks for continuous improvement. This is a fundamental requirement of quality improvement and a cornerstone of Lean organizations' design efforts. It also allows organizations to have predictability and reliability of work.

(Principle 7) Use visual control so no problems are hidden. Make the process as visible as possible so you can effectively identify process problems or compliance variance.

(Principle 8) Use only reliable, thoroughly tested technology. It is important to address process problems first and not assume that a technology will fix a broken process. If you are introducing a new technology, use Lean to ensure that it is implemented into work processes effectively.

Lean Methodology Advances an Organization Toward High Reliability

Through a foundation of problem prevention, problem solving, and continuous improvement, Lean allows processes to be developed that are reliable, safe, and supportive of people in the health care environment. Waste is reduced, quality is built into the work flow, and efficiencies follow. Those hospitals that provide the leadership and commitment to these methods are experiencing success, improving patient safety and supporting their staff in a learning environment.

SIX SIGMA

In addition to the Model for Improvement and Lean Methodology, organizations may want to consider using Six Sigma to achieve improvement. This is a multifaceted performance improvement strategy that focuses on making every step in a process as reliable as it can be. Six Sigma was heavily inspired by six preceding decades of quality improvement methodologies, such as Quality Control, Total Quality Management, and Zero Defects. Like its predecessors, Six Sigma asserts the following:

- Continuous effort to reduce variation in process outputs is key to success.

- Processes can be measured, analyzed, improved, and controlled.

- Succeeding at achieving sustained quality improvement requires commitment from the entire organization, particularly from top-level management.

The core of the Six Sigma methodology is a data-driven, systematic approach to problem solving, with a focus on customer impact. Statistical tools and analysis are often useful in the process. However, an acceptable Six Sigma project can be started with only rudimentary statistical tools.

Six Sigma has two key methodologies,[9] both inspired by W. Edwards Deming's Plan-Do-Study-Act Cycle. The first methodology, Define-Measure-Analyze-Improve-Control (DMAIC), is used to improve an existing process. The steps involved in DMAIC are as follows:

- *Define* the process improvement goals.

- *Measure* the current process and collect relevant data for future comparison.

- *Analyze* to verify relationship and causality of factors. Determine what the relationship is and attempt to ensure that all factors have been considered.

- *Improve* or optimize the process based on the analysis.

- *Control* to ensure that any variances are corrected before they result in defects.

The second methodology, Define-Measure-Analyze-Design-Verify (DMADV), is used to create highly reliable designs for new processes. The steps involved in DMADV are as follows:

- *Define* the goals of the design activity.

- *Measure* and identify critical qualities, process capabilities, and risk assessments.

- *Analyze* to develop and design alternatives, create high-level design, and evaluate design capability to select the best design.

- *Design* details, optimize the design, and plan for design verification. This phase may require simulations.

- *Verify* the design, set up pilot runs, implement the process, and hand over to process owners.

Six Sigma identifies several key roles for its successful implementation, as follows[10,11]:

- *Executive Leadership* is responsible for setting up a vision for Six Sigma implementation. They also empower the other role holders with the freedom and resources to explore new ideas for breakthrough improvements.

- *Champions* are responsible for the Six Sigma implementation across the organization in an integrated manner.

- *Master Black Belts*, identified by champions, act as in-house expert coaches for the organization on Six Sigma.

- *Black Belts* operate under Master Black Belts to apply Six Sigma methodology to specific projects.

- *Green Belts* are the employees who take up Six Sigma implementation along with their other job responsibilities. They operate under the guidance of Black Belts and support them in achieving the overall results.

- *Yellow Belts* are employees who have been trained in Six Sigma techniques as part of a corporatewide initiative but have not completed a Six Sigma project and are not expected to actively engage in quality improvement activities.

TOOLS FOR USE IN PERFORMANCE IMPROVEMENT

Key components to all the previously discussed improvement approaches are studying the process you want to improve, identifying areas of risk and waste, and determining opportunities for improvement. Two tools that can help with these efforts are discussed below.

FAILURE MODE AND EFFECTS ANALYSIS

Failure Mode and Effects Analysis (FMEA)[12] is a team-based, systematic, *proactive* technique used to prevent problems before they occur. It is used to analyze potential failures of systems, components, or functions and their effects. Each component is considered in turn with its possible modes of failure defined and the potential defects delineated.[13] It provides a look not only at what problems could occur but also at how severe the effects of the problems could be. FMEA is conducted with the assumption that no matter how knowledgeable or careful people are, failures will occur in some situations and may even be likely to occur. The focus is on *what* could allow the failure to occur, rather than *whom*. The FMEA technique is based on studied engineering principles and approaches to designing systems and processes. It has been successfully used in a number of industries, including the airline, automotive, and aerospace industries. Varying by the source consulted, FMEA can involve from as few as 4 to as many as 10 different steps. The approach described below has 8 key steps, as follows[12]:

1. Select a high-risk process and assemble a team.
2. Describe the process.
3. Brainstorm potential failure modes and determine their effects.
4. Prioritize failure modes.
5. Identify root causes of failure modes.
6. Redesign the process.
7. Analyze and test the new process.
8. Implement and monitor the redesigned process.

When conducting an FMEA, teams should answer some questions, including the following:

• What are the steps in the process? If it is an existing process, how does it currently occur and how should it occur? If it is a new process, how should it occur?

• How are the steps interrelated? (For example, are they sequential or do they occur simultaneously?)

• How is the process related to other health care processes?

• What tools should be used to diagram the process?

• What is the manner in which this process could fail? (When answering this question, team members should consider how people, materials, equipment, other processes and procedures, and the environment affect the process.)

• What are the potential effects of the identified failures? Effects of failures might be direct or indirect; long- or short-term; or likely or unlikely to occur. The severity of effects can vary considerably, from a minor annoyance to death or permanent loss of function. In this part of the process, team members should think through all the possible effects of a failure and list them for reference.

• What are the root causes of prioritized failure modes? What would have to go wrong for a failure like this to happen? What underlying weaknesses in the system might allow this to happen? What safeguards (for example, double checks) are present in the process? Are there any missing? If the process already contains safeguards, why might they not work to prevent the failure every time? If this failure occurred, why would the problem not be identified before it affected a patient?

By increasing staff members' understanding of the process under scrutiny, particularly from the perspective of their colleagues, undertaking an FMEA serves to enhance multidisciplinary teamwork and communication.[14]

ROOT CAUSE ANALYSIS

Another tool that can be helpful when further identifying and defining a problem or process to study is root cause analysis.[15,16] Root cause analysis (RCA) is a process for identifying the basic or causal factors that underlie variations in performance. Variations in performance can (and often do) produce unexpected and undesired adverse outcomes, including the occurrence or risk of a sentinel event.

Like FMEA, an RCA focuses primarily on systems and processes, not on the performance of a particular person. Through RCA, a team works to understand a process or processes, the causes or potential causes of variation, and process changes that make variation less likely to occur in the future. Root cause analysis is most commonly used *reactively* to probe the reason for a bad outcome or for failures that have already occurred. It can also be used to probe a near-miss event or as part of the FMEA process.

A thorough and credible root cause analysis has several steps. Many of the steps involved in RCA are similar to those in FMEA, and can be summarized as follows[13]:

1. Organize a team.
2. Define the problem.
3. Study the problem.
4. Determine what happened.
5. Identify the contributing factors.

6. Collect and assess data on proximate and underlying causes.

7. Design and implement interim changes.

8. Determine the root causes.

9. Explore and identify risk-reduction strategies.

10. Evaluate proposed actions.

11. Design, test, and implement improvements.

12. Evaluate and communicate the results of improvements.

By using root cause analysis to dig deep and discover the primary system issues causing error(s), organizations can target improvement efforts to reach the areas that will have the greatest impact on safety.

REFERENCES

1. Institute for Healthcare Improvement. How to Improve. (Updated: Aug 28, 2012.) Accessed Nov 1, 2012. http://www.ihi.org/knowledge/Pages/HowtoImprove/default.aspx.

2. Langley GL, et al. *The Improvement Guide: A Practical Approach to Enhancing Organizational Performance,* 2nd ed. San Francisco: Jossey-Bass; 2009.

3. The Joint Commission. Universal Protocol. Accessed Nov 1, 2012. http://www.jointcommission.org/standards_information/up.aspx.

4. Moen RD, Norman CL. Cycling back: Clearing up myths about the Deming cycle and seeing how it keeps evolving. *Quality Progress.* 2010;43(11):21–28.

5. Rogers E. *Diffusion of Innovations,* 4th ed. New York City: Free Press, 1995.

6. Likert JK. *The Toyota Way.* New York City: McGraw-Hill, 2003.

7. The Joint Commission. *Advanced Lean Thinking: Proven Methods to Reduce Waste and Improve Quality in Health Care.* Oak Brook, IL: Joint Commission Resources, 2008.

8. Spear S, Bowen HK. Decoding the DNA of the Toyota Production System. *Harv Bus Rev.* 1999;77(5):96–106.

9. De Feo JA, Barnard WW. *Juran Institute's Six Sigma Breakthrough and Beyond—Quality Performance Breakthrough Methods.* New York City McGraw-Hill, 2003.

10. Harry M, Schroeder R. *Six Sigma.* New York City: Random House, 2000.

11. Motorola University. Six Sigma Dictionary. Accessed Nov 1, 2012. http://www.motorola.com/web/Business/_Moto_University/_Documents/_Static_Files/Six_Sigma_Dictionary.pdf (accessed Jun. 14, 2012).

12. The Joint Commission. *Failure Mode and Effects Analysis in Health Care: Proactive Risk Reduction,* 3rd ed. Oak Brook, IL: Joint Commission Resources, 2010.

13. Vincent C. *Human Error Assessment and Reduction Technique, HEART Patient Safety.* Edinburgh: Elsevier, 2006.

14. Ashley L, et al. A practical guide to failure mode and effects analysis in health care: Making the most of the team and its meetings. *Jt Comm J Qual Patient Saf.* 2010;36(8):351–358.

15. Croteau RJ, editor. *Root Cause Analysis in Health Care: Tools and Techniques,* 4th ed. Oak Brook, IL: Joint Commission Resources, 2010.

16. US Department of Veterans Affairs, National Center for Patient Safety. Root Cause Analysis (RCA). Accessed Nov 1, 2012. http://www.patientsafety.gov/rca.html.

Chapter Thirteen

BUILDING AND SUSTAINING A LEARNING SYSTEM—FROM THEORY TO ACTION

Allan Frankel, MD; Michael Leonard, MD

INTRODUCTION

In 1994, in his sentinel article, "Errors in medicine," Lucian Leape wrote that health care must be redesigned to focus on reducing error and improving safety and reliability at the organizational and national level.[1] Since then, the health care industry has been unable to substantively accomplish this redesign work,[2,3] and health care today is neither reliable nor cost-effective.[4,5]

This chapter provides a simple and practical framework for redesigning health care at the unit level to achieve reliability and cost-effectiveness, combining concepts from human factors and organizational development with practical, clinical experience.

What may be surprising is that clinicians use the skills needed to apply this framework every day when they examine and treat patients. Clinicians treat patients by piecing together information from various sources, making diagnoses, and selecting treatments based on an understanding of the body's organ systems. Subsequently, they evaluate the treatment response and identify a delineated endpoint. These skills can be effectively applied to organizational improvement if clinicians' frame of reference is appropriately shifted so they see themselves as "guardians of the learning system" where they deliver care. As shown in Figure 13-1 (page 138), learning systems may be characterized as a cyclical process from defect identification through action to feedback and validation. They are dependent on effective leaders and teams, and the entire mechanism requires generous doses of psychological safety and a just culture.

To achieve safe and reliable operational excellence, physicians, nurses, pharmacists, and other health care personnel must become as familiar with the components of their department or unit as they are with the needs of their patients. Likewise, they must become as focused on the prevention of diseased or dysfunctional workplace processes as they are on the treatment of their patients. Fundamentally, health care professionals have to approach operational excellence with the same intensity and expertise that they bring to patient care. They must, in other words, become "organizational physicians."

ORGANIZATIONAL PHYSICIANS

Health care departments, units, and organizations—like patients—are unique, but they are also universally similar in that they have a set of basic organlike systems. These unit-level systems are describable, have observable characteristics when they are healthy, and show specific and nonspecific signs and symptoms when they are not. They are amenable to standardized treatments; they must be exercised to remain healthy; and as in humans, dysfunction in any one of the systems seriously degrades the health of the whole. These systems also require ongoing monitoring and periodic in-depth examination.

A health care unit has eight "organ systems," which can be divided into two main categories: Learning and Culture. Within the Learning category there are four organ systems:

1. The Reliable Process system
2. The Improvement system
3. The Measurement system
4. The Transparency system

Within the Culture category, there are also four organ systems:

1. The Leadership system
2. The Teamwork system

Figure 13-1. Cyclical Process of Learning Systems

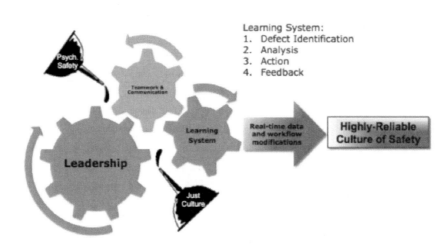

Learning System:
1. Defect Identification
2. Analysis
3. Action
4. Feedback

Source: Michael S. Woods, Pascal Metrics, Inc. Used with permission.

3. The Communication system

4. The Accountability system

In the next two sections, we take a closer look at these organ systems.

THE FOUR ORGANS OF LEARNING
The Reliable Process System

Consistency is appreciated everywhere—from an outstanding athlete who repeats a skill without defect to a service provider who repeatedly satisfies customers by delivering an excellent product. There are numerous hurdles to achieving reliable processes in health care. First, the fact that every patient is unique does not mean that every treatment must be unique, but we tend to conflate these ideas. Second, health care providers receive little to no instruction in process improvement,[6] human factors,[7] complexity theory,[8] or organizational management,[9] and so they do not realize the importance of, or how to achieve, reliable processes. Third, health care is complex. Simplifying it and reliably reproducing steps is seldom easy to achieve. Finally, physicians have historically resisted the development of standardized processes, seeing standardization as diminishing authority and autonomy.[10]

Ultimately, desired outcomes are more likely to be achieved if the steps to achieve them are minimized, simplified, easily reproduced, and reliably performed. Every unit should be consistently redesigning its processes to achieve these attributes. The units that do are likely to have the highest patient satisfaction scores, the happiest employees, and the best outcomes.

The Improvement System

As discussed in Chapter 12, Lean, Six Sigma, and the Model for Improvement are all improvement methods designed to help units achieve reliable and affordable processes. There are fundamental components in all these methods, and they are applied to a set of sequential actions. Each method requires baseline measurement, unit members that participate in small tests that change the activity in the unit, and measurement of the effects of change. Each method requires the stating of goals or aims that help to link the small tests that are performed with the overall aims to be achieved. None of this is rocket science. Effective improvement requires some basic skills and an open mind willing to consider change as a natural part of improvement.

Probably the most important part of a unit's improvement "organ system" is that everyone who works in the unit has at least a minimal understanding about tests of change[11] and that they are required to participate in some of these tests. Clinical acumen alone is no longer sufficient for practice in a clinical unit. Clinicians, as organizational physicians, must understand and have a common language for improvement.

The Measurement System

Every clinician understands the strength and vagaries of measurement. A radiologist reads an x-ray film and then quantifies the likely accuracy of his or her interpretation. Internists look at a few blood-pressure readings and make a decision about the efficacy of a drug treatment. In comparison to large double-blinded randomized trials, these measures are simple and few, but they are also adequate to make reasoned decisions. Unit performance can be measured in a similar manner. For example, a busy operating room performing 100 cases per day that wants to measure how effectively preoperative antibiotics are given prior to incision could look at 10 random operations as a baseline measure. These operations are likely more than adequate for a chart of performance over time, and if 9 out of 10 are performed adequately, the unit could document a 90% success rate for that week.

Fundamentally, measurement for improvement must be simple, expedient, and sufficient to make decisions—just like the measurement done in direct patient care. Small measurements over time, in the past ridiculed by primary researchers whose interests were creating new knowledge by collecting vast amounts of information in controlled trials, are now understood to be a powerful way of measuring how effectively we apply what is known.[12]

The Transparency System

Measuring, tracking, and highlighting processes and defects serve multiple purposes. The effort to do so identifies what leaders perceive as important and focuses provider and employee attention on topics that can improve reliability, help achieve strategic goals, and attain desired outcomes. It also extends beyond showcasing clinical activities and stresses the importance of culture. For example, units might measure the quality and frequency of briefings and debriefings. The units can set goals for these behaviors and measure the impact they have on daily care. One measure of briefings is to ask providers at the end of the day or procedure whether the briefing changed any of

their actions. The measurement of these cultural attributes must be transparent for them to be reliably performed. Such transparency underscores the value of the efforts and their importance to the unit's overall mission. Also, unit members are more likely to volunteer their effort and time, above what is mandatorily expected of them, when they feel they are participating in and shaping the world where they work. In fact, volunteering is a hallmark characteristic of successful organizations, and those organizations whose workers don't volunteer their time and efforts are likely doomed to mediocrity.[9]

THE FOUR ORGANS OF CULTURE
The Leadership System

Leadership in units is a distributed responsibility and applies to physicians, as well as other clinicians and administrators who have managerial responsibilities. For example, the surgeon in the operating room, the charge nurse on the floor, the internist or surgeon in the office practice, and the pharmacist leading medication rounds all assume the mantle of leadership. When they do, their first responsibility, and the hallmark of the leadership system, is that they become guardians of learning. They are responsible for safeguarding the four organs of learning—reliable process, improvement, measurement, and transparency. Leaders must be judged on how well they perform this function.

Learning is dependent on participants speaking up about their insights and concerns, so leaders must generate an environment of psychological safety,[13] in which concerns are easily discussed and made transparent. As discussed in Chapter 6, psychological safety describes an environment in which asking questions, requesting feedback, suggesting new ideas, and questioning things that seem out of place are welcomed and supported. Creating this environment is the job of leaders. High-quality, unit-based surveys are excellent methods for finding out whether leaders have created and nurtured psychological safety.

The Teamwork and Communication Systems

Teams are groups of individuals who, by planning forward, reflecting back, communicating clearly, and resolving conflict quickly, generate and maintain a common goal and an agreed-on game plan. There are discrete behaviors that support each of these actions and make up the teamwork and communication organ systems. As discussed in Chapter 6, briefings plan forward, facilitate a discussion about team goals, and help form the game plan as to what the team expects to unfold. Debriefings reflect back on an activity performed and are essential to improvement and learning. Accuracy of transmitted and received communications is dependent on structured communication techniques like SBAR (Situation, Background, Assessment, Recommendation)[14] and read-backs. Conflict resolution requires multiple techniques, but begins with the use of agreed-on terms to stop activity when perceived risk becomes too high or a team member can't link the team's actions to the game plan. These are "critical language" terms like "I need clarity" or "I'm concerned."

Although these behaviors are not conceptually difficult, it has been challenging to embed them in health care. Measuring them and highlighting their importance on process and debriefing boards such as those described below is a mechanism to support their use. Culture survey questions evaluate these teamwork and communication "organ systems" by asking questions about coordination between disciplines, the ability to speak up about concerns, conflict resolution, and the use of structured communications in handoffs.

The Accountability System

Simply put, individuals must be appropriately accountable for their actions, but should not be held accountable for actions beyond their control. The mechanisms to accomplish this have been described by Reason,[15] Marx,[16] Leonard and Frankel,[17] and Hickson et al.[18] As discussed in Chapter 3, when something goes wrong, the behaviors of the people involved should be assigned to one of five categories—Impaired Judgment, Malicious Action, reckless Action, Risky Action, or Unintentional Error (*see* Figure 13-2 on page 141). After a reflective jury agrees on the designation into which the behaviors fall, the response must be aimed, first and foremost, at decreasing risk, and second, at maintaining the integrity of the learning system. In other words, unit members should perceive the organizational response as fair and just. There are exceptions where "groupthink" skews behavior by a whole group, in which case leaders must be aware of these situations and manage them. For example, the death of a new mother on an obstetrics unit led to the discovery that a standard postcesarean (C-section) order was for morphine in 2-milligram increments up to 30 milligrams total, at the discretion of the RN administering the medication. Thirty milligrams is a huge dose of morphine, yet hundreds of obstetrics RNs and dozens of obstetricians at this hospital had slowly deviated toward this standard order set. Explanations extended from the rationale that RNs had the skill to make the right decision to the belief that because pregnant mothers have a larger intravascular volume and pregnancy-induced edema, they needed larger doses of opiates to relieve pain. In retrospect, the orders decreased the number of phone calls between RNs and physicians and simply made the care easier for both parties, but at significantly increased risk to patients. The solution was to require the RN to call the physician after administering 10 milligrams of morphine to discuss the patient's care plan. That one step decreased the average total morphine dose post–C-section from 17 mg to 11 mg without any increase in patient pain scores. Transparency of process, outcomes, and error assists here. Processes should be based first on best evidence and then on consensus. The discussions that generate agreement about the appropriate steps for a process are likely to keep the unit from deviating too much from known good practice. Measurement, goal setting, and transparency of process and defects then help the group to stay on course. Process measurements identify the reliability of the current state while goal setting establishes expectation about improvement.

When things do go wrong, as they inevitably will in the complex world of health care, the evaluation of the event should not be inordinately influenced by the outcome or by pressure from the public or the media.

ASSESSING AND TREATING THE ORGANIZATION

Organizational physicians should examine organization units using an approach that is similar to examining patients: generating an initial impression, conducting a history that includes a review of organ systems, and finally performing a physical examination and obtaining laboratory data. The following sections walk through this type of examination and demonstrate how it can improve unit health, productivity, and reliability.

The Initial Impression

When generating an initial impression of a unit's eight organ systems, we can see whether the systems reflect a healthy and

Figure 13-2. The Fair Evaluation and Response Chart

HOW TO USE THIS CHART: This chart should be used to categorize an individual caregiver's actions, not groups or systems. Evaluate each factor that influenced the caregiver's actions separately . When determining accountability, consider the context in which the action occurred.

IMPAIRED JUDGMENT	MALICIOUS ACTION
The caregiver's thinking was impaired - by illegal or legal substances - by cognitive impairment - by severe psychosocial stressors	The caregiver wanted to cause harm.
• Discipline is warranted if illegal substances were used. • The caregiver's mindset and performance should be evaluated to determine whether a temporary work suspension would be helpful. • Help should be actively offered to the caregiver.	• Discipline and/or legal proceedings are warranted. • The caregiver's duties should be suspended immediately.

2. Second, use best judgment to categorize each action as either Reckless, Risky or Unintentional based on the definitions in the Chart. The categorization determines the general level of culpability and possible disciplinary actions, however these general categories require further analysis as below prior to making a final decision.

RECKLESS ACTION	RISKY ACTION	UNINTENTIONAL ERROR
The caregiver knowingly violated a rule and/or made a dangerous or unsafe choice. The decision appears to be self serving and to have been made with little or no concern about risk.	The caregiver made a potentially unsafe choice. Their evaluation of relative risk appears to be erroneous.	The caregiver made or participated in an error while working appropriately and in the patients' best interests
• The caregiver is accountable and needs re-training. Discipline may be warranted • The caregiver should participate in teaching others the lessons learned.	• The caregiver is accountable and should receive coaching. • The caregiver should participate in teaching others the lessons learned.	• The caregiver is not accountable. • The caregiver should participate in investigating why the error occurred and teach others about the results of the investigation.

3. Third, perform a Substitution Test by evaluating (usually be directly asking) whether other individuals with similar skills and in a similar situation might find themselves performing a similar action under similar circumstances. If yes, then there are systematic issues leading to this situation, and individual accountability is less. If no, then the individual is fully accountable.

The system supports reckless action and requires fixing. The caregiver is probably less accountable for the action, and system leaders share in the accountability.	The system supports risky action and requires fixing. The caregiver is probably less accountable for the action, and system leaders share in the accountability.	The system supports error and requires fixing. The system's leaders are accountable and should apply error-proofing improvements.

4. Fourth, evaluate whether the individual has a history of unsafe or problematic acts. If they do, this may influence decisions about the appropriate responsibilities for the individual i.e. they may be in the wrong job. Organizations should have a reasonable and agreed upon statute of limitations for taking these actions into account.

This figure provides one example of an approach to ensuring a fair and just response to errors, adverse event, or near misses.

Source: Michael Leonard and Allan Frankel, Pascal Metrics, Inc. Used with permission.

robust unit. The healthiest units, those most likely to achieve safe and reliable operational excellence, will have large areas of dedicated wall space for bulletin boards that focus on three specific aspects of unit work; processes, defects, and outcomes. These bulletin boards demonstrate the transparency "organ system" at work and showcase the activities of and interplay between the other organ systems.

Just as the physician's initial impression of a human patient is the summation of the interplay among the body's organs, so too is the initial impression of a unit. These boards are physical manifestations of excellent leadership, teamwork, and learning. They indicate that processes are measured, and that transparency is the order of the day. They suggest that there is healthy interplay between the unit-level organ components.

Following is a brief discussion of the three types of bulletin boards. (Figure 13-3, below, visually demonstrates this concept.)

Process Bulletin Board

As discussed in Chapter 4, reliable processes stem from using the fewest actions to achieve a consistent outcome. Such processes also minimize variation in each action to ensure that output leads to a high level of quality. To achieve this consistency and high quality and apply improvements when needed, a unit must conduct improvement tests, simply measure test results, and make these efforts abundantly transparent to all who work in or travel through the unit. Process boards measure the percentage of time a bundled set of actions occurs and includes the target goal identified for that process.

Process boards can measure a variety of activities. Some will align with senior leadership strategic programs; some with issues specific to a particular unit; and others will show-case efforts chosen by frontline providers. The boards are an ideal medium to focus attention on bundles of steps that can be purposefully designed for simplicity, reproducibility, and ultimately reliability. They can also be used as the medium

Figure 13-3. Transparency Bulletin Boards

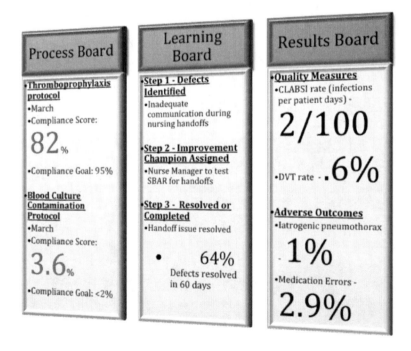

This figure shows the three types of bulletin boards that should be present on a unit to highlight and communicate about various aspects of unit work.

Source: Allan Frankel, Pascal Metrics, Inc. Used with permission.

to inform providers of how effectively change is being implemented, as they are ideally suited to make performance measures transparent.

In addition to serving as a communication medium process boards can also serve as a marketing technique that continually highlights what unit leadership perceives as important. These boards make improvement efforts widely visible, and then track unit success. The value of process boards is that they indicate to personnel what they need to think about on a particular day and in a particular moment. For example, in an ambulatory clinic, measured processes might include the number of patients seen each day, the percentage of outside phone calls answered within 60 seconds, and, during flu season, the percentage of patients who are asked about, and, appropriately given, a flu shot.

Process boards must be carefully designed to maximize and simplify their message. The best bulletin boards show simple large numbers, as suggested by Figure 13-4, below. Any supporting run charts and bar charts can be placed on secondary boards in less public areas or maintained on computers or in logbooks. The process boards should indicate how well the processes are being done over some period of time, and also clearly outline the target goal.

Process boards can help align the perceptions and perspectives of senior leadership and frontline workers, which are often quite divergent. As an example of this divergence, the lowest scores in hospital attitudinal surveys are usually related to the perception of senior leadership by frontline providers. More effective communication is the first remedy for this, and the process board, along with the defect and outcomes boards discussed below, is the place to begin.

Learning Boards

The learning board, sometimes called the debriefing or defect board, showcases frontline providers' concerns and the actions being taken to address them. The concerns should be collected during debriefings and also from sources such as spontaneous reporting systems, audits, and quality

Figure 13-4. A Process Bulletin Board

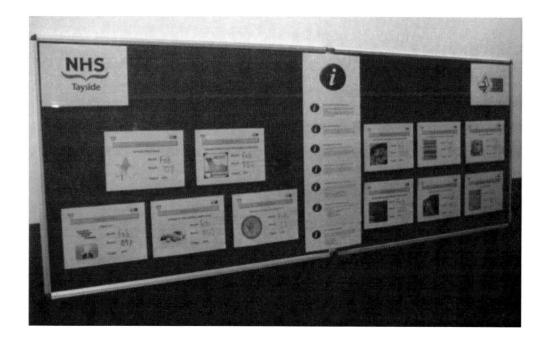

This figure illustrates an effective process bulletin board, which highlights the important aspects of improvement work, including current performance and the target goal.

Source: Arun Chaudhri, Acute Medicines Unit, Tayside Hospital, Dundee, Scotland. Used with permission.

metrics, and all should be integrally woven into the unit's clinical work *(see* Chapter 6).

Conducted routinely—that is, daily or after procedures—debriefings provide managers with the content for the debriefing board and support continuous learning and action. The learning board can also include patient concerns. The influence patients have must be obvious, transparent, and loudly communicated. (*See* Chapter 9 for more information about the importance of patient influence.)

The learning board should be divided into 3 parts. (*See* Figure 13-5 on page 145). After each debriefing, issues identified should be written on cards and the cards placed onto the first part of the board. All cards should be placed on the board with the exception of those that blame or target specific individuals, which should be managed separately (*See* Chapter 6) Some organizations divide the cards into categories, such as Equipment, Patient Flow, and so on. The most advanced debriefing boards have categories about cultural and teamwork issues such as briefings, debriefings, and perceptions of risk.

A concern is moved to the second part of the learning board when an individual or team is assigned responsibility to address or solve the concern. The card is moved to the third part of the board when the issue has been resolved. Seeing the movement across the board is empowering. Like the process board, the learning board is a communication medium and also a form of marketing. It showcases that frontline concerns are important and that the concerns are acted on and addressed. Although issues could be tracked in a logbook or computer and the findings periodically reported, these methods do not seem to effectively push the data into the work environment. They also don't adequately support the transparency organ system. The process of identifying defects and acting on them is a fundamental job of unit management and its engagement with frontline staff. The movement of the concerns across the defect board is a visible testimonial to effective management and at the same time empowers frontline workers to speak up about their concerns because they see them being acted on. Note that the willingness of unit members to speak up is also directly related to the level of psychological safety that exists in that unit.

The Results Board
The results board showcases a unit's outcomes. These include outcomes related to the unit's quality of care and

also the unit's adverse event rates. As in the process and learning boards, the results board fosters transparent communication, advertising, and more. The metrics included on the board identify the overall departmental goals and strategy. By showing the adverse event rates, the board highlights the importance of ongoing risk evaluation.

The results board also showcases the strategic interests of senior management, and when they visit a unit, such as during WalkRounds, they should meet with frontline staff in front of the process, learning, and results boards. In so doing, they are much more likely to effectively engage frontline employees in discussions about topics of importance to the unit and organization. It is also more likely that everyone will come away from the interaction with a unified sense of goals and challenges.

The History: Review of Systems
After the initial impression, organizational physicians must deepen their insight by taking a history and then performing a review of systems in which questions are focused on each organ's function. When physicians perform a review of systems on human patients, they ask specific organ-attributable questions. For example, they ask about shortness of breath, palpitations, bowel habits, and gait to query the function of the respiratory, cardiovascular, gastrointestinal, and musculoskeletal systems, respectively. A survey of unit culture and interviews of unit staff are the equivalent to this physical system assessment and require that organizational physicians understand what each organ does and how it works.

This review of systems is an evaluation of unit culture. In health care, we have tended to think of culture as the soft side of the equation, as opposed to the hard-edged medical world so often filled with numbers and facts. Nothing could be further from reality. Culture is measurable, understandable, and malleable (*see* Chapter 2, "Assessing and Improving Safety Culture"). The colloquial description of culture as "the way we do things around here" is succinct but functionally inadequate. Schein defines culture more robustly as having three tiers—the first tier consists of the visible attributes, including how people interact with each other; the second, the espoused values (mission and value statements); and the third, the hidden values, the often unspoken and sometimes subconscious drivers of behavior.[19] As stated, as hidden values diverge, the likelihood of

Figure 13-5. The Learning Board

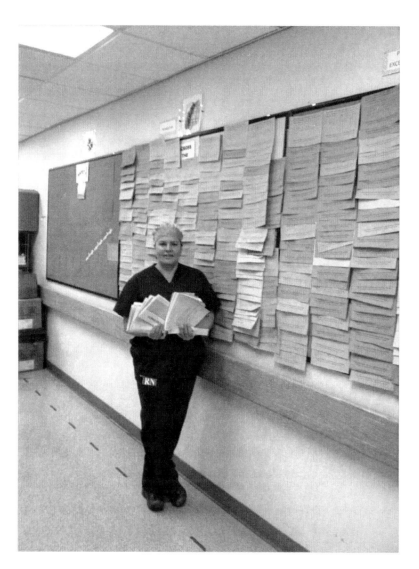

This figure illustrates an organization's learning board on which providers note concerns and they are acted upon and resolved.

Source: Melissa Fritz, RN, Anderson Mercy Hospital, Catholic Health Partners, Cincinnati. Used with permission.

operational excellence declines.[20] For example, nurses and physicians may be polite to each other (the visible attribute) and be able to recite the espoused value of "patient-centered care." However, if the nurses complain that the physicians hastily walk past the nursing station on the way to see their patients in an effort to shorten the time they round, resulting in nurses not knowing the daily game plan for a patient, then the hidden value—physician-centered care—is clearly at odds with patient-centered care. The physicians may have good reason for hurrying, such as the need to see the other patients waiting in their offices or the emergency room. Nevertheless, the tension generated undermines morale and learning.

Attitudinal surveys and interviews, and the conversations that arise from the results, are an exceptionally good way to evaluate and understand the three layers of culture.

The insights may then be applied using tests of change from the improvement organ system, and the results shown on a process board.

The Physical Exam

The physical exam, which is similar to the patient's physical exam, allows an organizational physician to study the geographic layout of a unit; the way employees interact with each other and with patients; how patients move through the unit; the interfaces with other units during handoffs and when transporting patients; the methods for sharing information; and the approach to storing and accessing equipment. Performing the exam may be as simple as a walk through the unit to see the physical layout; sitting quietly in the unit nursing station and observing interactions; or being treated to a tour of the unit, with managers or frontline providers describing what works—and what doesn't—in each area. Questions about factors that lead to rework, walking extra distances, frustration in finding stored equipment, help in further delineating issues. This examination identifies Schein's "visible attributes"[19] and elucidates the functional strengths and limitations in the unit. The processes in the unit must be tailored to build on the strengths and work around the limitations that are evident in the physical exam. All too often, processes accentuate weakness and do not take advantage of strengths, such as when the safeguard to prevent an error relies predominantly on providing a note to remind busy clinicians to be vigilant, as opposed to, say, a constraint or forcing function that would help them do the right thing.

Diagnosis and Treatment

As mentioned earlier, health care providers learn to make diagnoses based on the patient's symptoms and signs. Often patients will have multiple diagnoses, as when a patient's slow walk is a result of arthritis and congestive heart failure. Expert clinicians learn to distinguish the influence of multiple organ dysfunctions on the patient's signs and symptoms. Similarly, a dysfunctional unit may be a result of multiple issues, such as inadequate leadership and inadequate learning. Because the health care field has not trained units or leaders in the manner described in this chapter, we find that many units have the equivalent of complex medical problems.

These problems can be solved. For example, if the diagnosis shows that effective leadership is wanting, then leaders can be trained. The development of learning systems and promotion and safeguarding of psychological safety are teachable skills. Current health care leaders tend to manifest these skills along a spectrum: those who know what to do, those who mean well but haven't been trained, and those who shouldn't lead. Leaders who "get it" realize the value of team behaviors that generate learning, and support and participate in them. They lead briefings that clarify the game plan, and they lead or support debriefings where defects come to light.[20]

Teamwork behaviors become evident and consistent when the unit's participants understand their value, when the behaviors are observed and their quality measured, and when those measures are specific.[21] If the diagnosis is that some aspect of teamwork is lacking, then a team behavior such as "briefings" can be added to the process board and the frequency and quality of the briefings measured.

The use or nonuse of a learning board can also highlight good or poor unit health. If the board exists but is not populated, that is a sign of disease to be evaluated. The underlying cause may be lack of psychological safety or the perception that no effective actions will be taken to address concerns. Each of these causes is amenable to treatment. Sharing the plan and inviting team members to speak up during every briefing models psychological safety. Acting on concerns is a function of understanding improvement methods and measurement. Units should have skills in improvement methods such as Lean, Six Sigma, and Rapid Cycle Improvement, to apply to the concerns of frontline providers and to move the debriefing cards across the three sections of the learning board, as described earlier. The speed of movement and the percentage of concerns acted on are measures of managerial and leadership competence in applying improvements to the unit.

Doubts about organizational fairness arise when things go wrong and unit members perceive the organizational response to be unjust. If the diagnosis is that there is concern about organizational fair play, then the treatment is to transparently use the Fair Evaluation and Response Chart (Figure 13-2) to demonstrate that there is a fair and consistent process to evaluate errors, adverse events, and near misses.[17] Training in use of the chart in simulated situations, with participation and open commitment by senior leadership, provides a powerful mechanism to build the accountability and trust that are essential to support and drive organizational learning.

SUMMARY

Organizational change for the better is possible if health care providers, particularly physician leaders, come to understand that they have a responsibility that runs parallel to, and ultimately improves the quality of, the care of patients. It is their responsibility to become guardians and keepers of organizational learning systems. For this to happen, departments must be viewed using the schema of organ components described, and the health of each organ component evaluated. Treatment, or the appropriate allocation of resources, should be based on the findings of a history and physical exam of each unit. Care should be taken to ensure that resources are not allocated solely to projects, such as fixing the medication delivery system, but also to the components that comprise the units' body and soul—its state of culture and learning. As in patients, one unhealthy organ system is often enough to strip away all evidence of robust health. Yet, some patients compensate remarkably well despite significant limitations. The job of the organizational physician, which characterizes almost everyone who works in a clinical care unit, is to examine and diagnose unit-level malaise, and to then participate in fixing it and ensuring that it doesn't return. Outstanding leadership is needed, and participation by all is mandatory. Fortunately, all these skills necessary for habitual excellence and safe, reliable care are teachable and can be readily applied to great benefit.

REFERENCES

1. Leape LL. Error in medicine. *JAMA*. 1994 Dec 21;272(23):1851–1857.
2. Landrigan CP, et al. Temporal trends in rates of patient harm resulting from medical care. *N Engl J Med*. 2010 Nov 25;363(22):2124-2134.
3. Classen DC, et al. 'Global Trigger Tool' shows that adverse events in hospitals may be ten times greater than previously measured. *Health Aff (Millwood)*. 2011;30(4):1–9.
4. Porter ME, Teisberg EO. *Redefining Health Care: Creating Value-Based Competition on Results*. Boston: Harvard Business School Press, 2006.
5. Anderson GF, Frogner BK. Health spending in OECD countries: Obtaining value per dollar. *Health Aff (Millwood)*. 2008;7(6):1718–1727.
6. Langley GL, et al. *The Improvement Guide: A Practical Approach to Enhancing Organizational Performance*, 2nd ed. San Francisco: Jossey-Bass, 2009.
7. Salvendy G. *Handbook of Human Factors and Ergonomics*, 2nd ed. New York City: Wiley, 1997.
8. Weick KE, Sutcliffe KM. *Managing the Unexpected: Resilient Performance in an Age of Uncertainty*, 2nd ed. San Francisco: Jossey-Bass, 2007.
9. Berry LL, Seltman KD. *Management Lessons from Mayo Clinic Inside One of the World's Most Admired Service Organizations*. New York City: McGraw-Hill, 2008.
10. Amalberti R, et al. Five system barriers to achieving ultrasafe health care. *Ann Intern Med*. 2005 May 3;142(9):756–764.
11. Leonard M, Frankel A, Simmonds T, editors: *Achieving Safe and Reliable Healthcare: Strategies and Solutions*. Chicago: Health Administration Press, 2004.
12. Davidoff F, et al.; SQUIRE Development Group. Publication guidelines for quality improvement studies in health care: Evolution of the SQUIRE project. *BMJ*. 2009 Jan 19;338:a3152.
13. Edmondson A. Psychological safety and learning behavior in work teams. *Administrative Science Quarterly*. 1999;44(2):350–383.
14. Leonard M, Graham S, Bonacum D. The human factor: The critical importance of effective teamwork and communication in providing safe care. *Qual Saf Health Care*. 2004;13 Suppl 1:i85–90.
15. Reason J. *Managing the Risks of Organizational Accidents*. Aldershot, UK: Ashgate, 1997.
16. Marx D. *Patient Safety and the "Just Culture": A Primer for Health Care Executives*. New York City: Columbia University, 2001.
17. Leonard MW, Frankel A. The path to safe and reliable healthcare. *Patient Educ Couns*. 2010;80(3):288–292.
18. Hickson GB, et al. Balancing systems and individual accountability in a safety culture. In The Joint Commission: *From Front Office to Front Line: Essential Issues for Health Care Leaders*, 2nd ed. Oak Brook, IL: Joint Commission Resources, 2011, 1–35
19. Schein EH. *Organizational Culture and Leadership: A Dynamic View*, 2nd ed. San Francisco: Jossey-Bass, 1992.
20. Argyris C. *Organizational Traps: Leadership, Culture, Organizational Design*. London: Oxford University Press, 2010.
21. Kozlowski SW, et al. Effects of training goals and goal orientation traits on multidimensional training outcomes and performance adaptability. *Organ Behav Hum Decis Process*. 2001;85(1):1–31.

Index

S

bulletin boards on units
    learning (defect) boards, 142, 143–144, 145, 146
    process boards, 142–143
    results boards, 142, 144
environment, assessment of, 146
organizational physicians, 137–138, 139, 140, 144, 146, 147
organlike systems, 137–140
reliability and cost-effectiveness and, 137–138, 147
Universal Protocol for Preventing Wrong Site, Wrong Procedure, Wrong Person Surgery™, 57–58, 126
University of Missouri Health Care *forYOU Team*, 86

V

Value-Based Purchasing program, v
Value Stream and Value Stream Map, 129–131
Verbal orders and read-back requirement, 62
Veterans Health Administration surgical safety initiative, 15
Virginia Mason Production System, vi
Vocabulary national standards, 104
Volunteering, 139

W

WalkRounds
    benefits of, 15, 44, 46, 125
    case examples
      Brigham and Women's Hospital WalkRounds program, 44, 45, 51
      National Health Service of England, South West region WalkRounds, 46, 47
      Sunnybrook Health Center WalkRounds program, 46, 48–49

CUSP model and, 65
development of concept of, 44
organization culture, gathering information about during, 2
purpose of and process for, 4, 15, 43–44, 45, 46, 49–52
    closing statements, 50
    debriefing, 50–51
    documentation of discussions, 44, 50
    feedback, 51–52
    measurement of effectiveness of, 52
    opening statements, 49, 50
    preparation for, 46
    questions to prompt discussion, 44, 46, 49–50
    reporting, 51
    scheduling, 46
    tracking information, 49
    where to conduct, 46, 49
Waste elimination, 126, 129, 132–133
Whiteboards, 64, 93
Work-arounds, 40, 109, 128
Work flow, 3, 35–38, 39, 40, 125, 126
World Health Organization (WHO) Surgical Safety Checklist, 57–58
Wrist bands, 107

Y

Yellow Belts (Six Sigma), 133

Z

Zero Defects, 133